Health, Hazard and the Higher Risk Traveller

by

Iain B. McIntosh, BA(Hons), MBChB, DGM RCP, DRCoG

illustrated by

Valerie A McIntosh

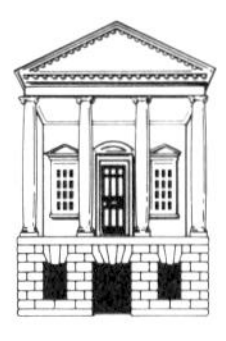

Quay Publishing

Quay Publishing Limited
7.1.9 Cameron House, White Cross
South Road, Lancaster, LA1 4XQ

British Library Cataloguing in Publication Data
A catalogue record for this book is available from the British Library

ISBN 1 85642 081 7

Printed in the United Kingdom by Bell and Bain, Glasgow

Contents

Introduction vii

Chapter

1 The travel health clinic 1

2 Poor hygiene and disease 23

3 The stress of modern travel 35

4 Travel phobias 47

5 Travel sickness 62

6 The child traveller 73

7 The woman traveller 86

8 The elderly traveller 101

9 The disabled and handicapped traveller 120

10 Health hazards and water sports abroad 131

11 High altitude, high risk travel 145

12 Expedition medicine 157

Appendix I 169

Appendix II 171

Appendix III 173

Appendix IV 175

Index 177

INTRODUCTION

Tourists of all ages travel across Europe and round the Mediterranean on package holidays. The more intrepid respond to the lure of distant places taking 'the holiday of a lifetime'. Transatlantic crossings and antipodean visits to distant relatives are commonplace. The young adventurer journeys to the far ends of the earth, explores the world's high places and undertakes risky sports and adventures in exotic climes. All those who venture abroad are exposed to travel-induced illness and some risk life and limb on international visits.

The majority return invigorated after a break from humdrum routine. Many resist the vagaries of foreign food, transport and adverse climates but some succumb to temperature extremes, local diseases and contaminated food and water supplies. At best, this may merely spoil a day or two of the holiday. Illness and trauma can, however, ruin the vacation. Ill-health may necessitate consultation with local doctors, exposure to the variable facilities of foreign hospitals and involve the family doctor on the return from the holiday. The unfortunate few may never recover from travel-acquired illness.

Anticipation of potential travel problems; identification of the higher-risk traveller; appropriate prophylaxis; relevant counselling and targeted health education can minimise travel risk. The GP-based travel health clinic is well placed to meet the demands of the international traveller. Doctor and practice nurse can provide a service which may help the individual avoid undue stress and illness on vacation.

Some travellers are at greater risk than others. Destination, transport mode, type of holiday and current medical status should all be considered in risk assessment. The very young, the old and disabled, the pregnant, the adventurer, watersports enthusiasts and high altitude climbers are at special risk of suffering from travel-induced illness. Many intending travellers suffer from travel phobia and some will be affected by travel sickness. Most are exposed to translocation and transportation-induced stress.

Travel risk, travel health assessment and management of potential problems are considered in the following chapters. The value of standardised health questionnaires and check lists is considered and specimen instruction leaflets are offered as aide-memoires for individuals about to embark on foreign travel.

The last few decades have seen an explosion in international travel with people of all ages regularly travelling outwith the UK, see Table 1. A mere four million passengers were transported by the world's airlines in 1948 compared to over 400 million today.

There is remarkably little in the literature regarding attack rates of travel-induced disease and its impact on general practice. Much of the published data has come from the Communicable Diseases (Scotland) Unit (CDSU) at Ruchill Hospital, Glasgow (Cossar, 1990). Since 1973 it has organised a survey of travellers returning to Scotland

Table Intro.1: Growth in international travel

	1949	1960	1970	1990
	M	M	M	M
Total numbers of international tourists	26	72	201	429
Total numbers of air travellers throughout the world	31	106	386	460
Total visits abroad by United Kingdom residents	1.7	6	11.8	31*
	(%)	(%)	(%)	(%)
Visits by United Kingdom residents (European destinations: rest of world)	92:8	94:6	89:11	84:16
Mode of travel used by United Kingdom residents (sea: air)	–	60:40	43:57	30:70
Proportion of package holiday visits abroad by United Kingdom residents	–	30	30	41*

* 1989 figures for UK residents
Printed by permission of Scottish Medicine

Some 14,000 people have participated with 37% reporting illness, mostly of an alimentary nature, while they were away (Figure 1). Many of these (14 percent) required the additional attention of a GP on their return and some required hospital admission (Reid, 1986). Travel-induced illness is an added burden on professional time and NHS resources.

In 1986 one in three travel brochures gave no health advice (Reid, 1986) and information provided by others was often inconsistent and inadequate. In one study, of the 48% of travellers who sought health advice, 35% reported later travel illness. The highest attack rate (45%) occurred in those receiving advice from the doctor – perhaps people

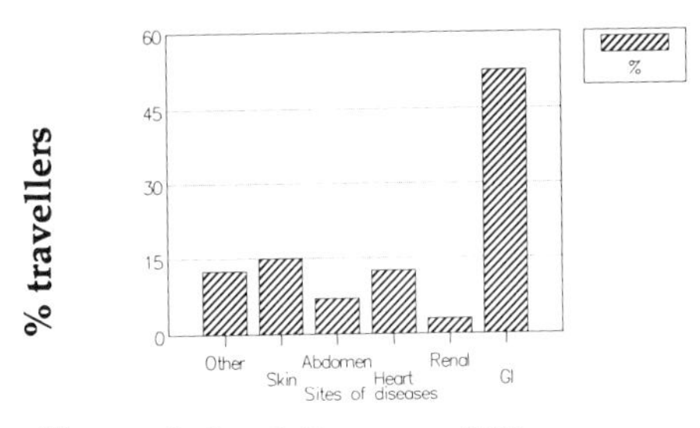

Figure Intro.1 Survey of illness affecting travellers over 65yrs of age

already suffering from pre-existing disease. It is known that GPs often recommend inappropriate and unnecessary vaccination to potential travellers but there is evidence that travellers would prefer to obtain pre-travel health advice from their own doctor (Cossar 1992).

A recent survey (McIntosh 1991) suggests higher attack rates in the old and illness in the elderly may be more severe and even life threatening (see Figure Intro.1). There is a paucity of data on treatment abroad and hospital admission in general but the older groups may have a higher admission rate (see Figure Intro.2).

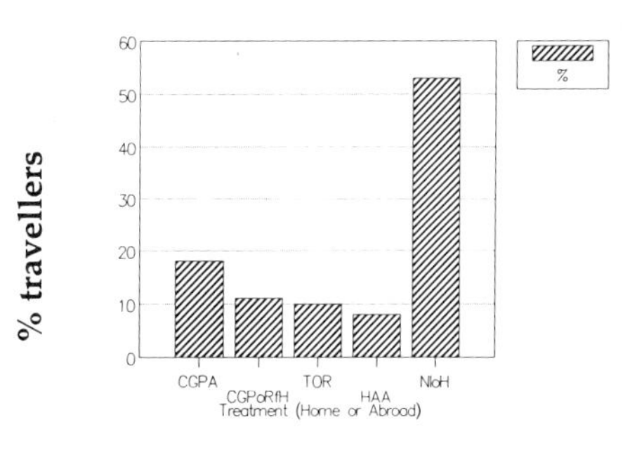

CGPA= Consult GP abroad
CGPoRfH= Consult GP on return from holiday
TOR=Travellers own remedy
HAA=Hospital admission abroad
NIoH=Not ill on holiday

Figure Intro.2 Responses to travellers' illness

D' A Paixao *et al* have recently observed that the main cause of travellers' death overseas is no longer infection but cardiovascular, with those aged 60 years plus, the most represented group (D'A Paixao, 1991). They suggest that there are health grounds for judicious consideration to be given to aged travellers' proposed travels.

With deterioration in immune response, the presence of pre-existing disease, renal dysfunction and the possibility of metabolic disorder, older travellers may not only be at greater risk of incurring disease abroad but are more likely to require professional assistance and hospitalisation.

Preparing for a healthy holiday

With the approach of the holiday season people gleefully pack suntan lotion and sandals and take off for a holiday in the sun, often with remarkably little preparation or thought for health and hygiene hazards which may be found at the chosen resort. Most will be heading for the polluted waters of the Mediterranean but each year increasing numbers venture further afield and expose themselves to exotic illnesses.

Cosseted by the National Health Service and accustomed to UK hygiene standards they fly off abroad, risking life and limb, sometimes with scant or dubious medical insurance.

Malignant falciparum malarial cases in the United Kingdom leapt from 326 in 1980 to over 779 in 1991. Malaria should always be borne in mind with ill tourists who are also suffering increasingly from diseases such as hepatitis A, polio and typhoid infections (Figure Intro.3).

Travel agents provide little relevant pre-travel information and many people are referred to their GPs for advice (Gorman 1992). Only the financial return ensures that they encourage insurance cover which may well prove inadequate when a medical emergency arises.

The quality of service offered by harassed family doctors varies widely, from a full advice and vaccination package to unenthusiastic, bland reassurance. Reluctant GPs are not wholly to blame for the situation for the majority of tourists return home unharmed. Accurate advice on vaccination and malaria prophylaxis can be difficult to obtain, with differing opinions advocated by different tropical medicine centres.

Appropriate prophylaxis becomes ever more complex for travellers to Asia and Africa. At the very least doctors should direct patients to the Department of Health publication called 'The Travellers' Guide to Health', an excellent booklet which also spells out the reciprocal arrangements the UK has with other EC countries. These arrangements are a variable feast even when one is the possessor of the crucial Form E111, which has to be obtained from the Department of Social Security at least one month in advance of the holiday.

Table Intro.2 Factors which can affect the traveller's health

- Temperature extremes:
  - High temperature risk
  - Low temperature risk
- Humidity
- Altitude
- Disturbances in circadian rhythm
- Air travel
- Sea/land/air transportation
- Cultural shock
- Environmental stress
- Communication problems
- Travel fatigue
- Physical stress
- Enforced immobility
- Risk of disease
- Trauma

British Airways recognise the gap in proficient advice and protection for travellers and has set up the Medical Advisory Service for Travellers Abroad (MASTA). Their aim is to cover the country with travel centres in association with group health centres and hospital units.

Provision of travel vaccinations can be an additional source of income for GPs and may prove a welcome addition to income subject, however, to proposed Government contractual changes. GPs can offer an effective service and it is certainly in their best interest to have patients return to the UK free from imported morbidity.

Occasionally, patients return from holiday with horrific tales of sudden illness. Emergency treatment may result in hospitalisation in a unit with poor hygienic standards, scant access to medication and gross overcrowding. In Asia, beds are crowded together, wards can be mud-floored and the water and energy supplies may be intermittent.

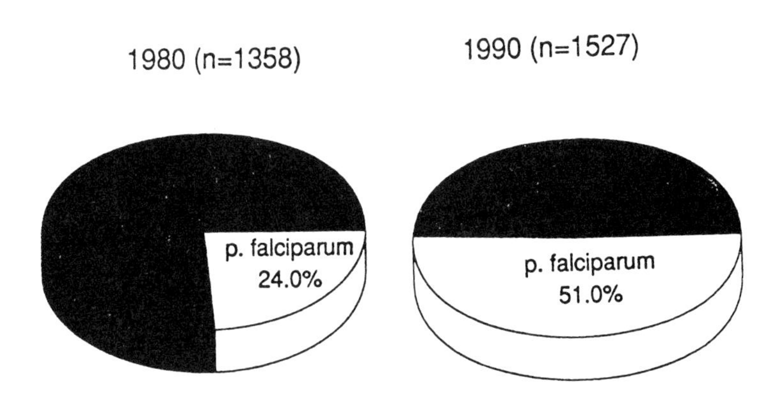

Figure Intro.4: Malaria notifications recorded in the UK

Case History Intro: 1

A female patient of mine was struck down suddenly by debilitating diarrhoea and vomiting in the city of Tashkent. She received prompt medical attention and was sped from her hotel by ambulance to a local infectious disease unit. The location of this hospital remained unknown to the rest of the travel group who had to continue on their tour without her. She was isolated in a small ward where no one spoke English. On arrival, she was stripped naked and hosed down in a sluice room. Later, she was given intravenous infusion with deteriorated, re-usable rubber and glass-giving apparatus and then dosed regularly with Mist. Trisil. She emerged from isolation cured of her diarrhoea but psychologically the worse for wear.

Patients are often lulled into a sense of false security having taken out insurance cover, but they forget that when abroad they can find themselves many miles or even days from good medical aid. Storm and flood, impossible terrain, avalanche and landslide, variable roads and communications, plus the barrier of language can make a mockery of the best of medical insurance. Even in Europe in the ski season, tourists can find themselves admitted to small isolated hospitals.

Alpine hospital units can be poorly prepared to deal with medical events other than orthopaedic emergency.

Case History Intro: 2

An elderly patient enjoying a ski-holiday, mistimed a slalom turn, landed heavily on his back and developed a pneumothorax. He was admitted urgently to a small orthopaedic unit in the Savoie Alps where x-rays were misinterpreted and his medical condition was mis-diagnosed. Only prompt air evacuation returned him to sound UK medical care. With costs of well over £1,000 an hour for helicopter evacuation when this is available, medical insurance cover can very quickly prove inadequate.

Any visit to the United States must carry maximal insurance cover – a fact which is still not appreciated by many elderly people who visit relatives in Canada and in the States each year.

It often falls to the family doctor to acquaint the traveller of other hazards which they may experience. For example, a road traffic accident during a safari in Africa, or even when crossing the road in Nairobi, may result in a blood transfusion, exposing the patient to a 50% possibility of acquiring AIDS.

In the Baltic states and the new Federal Russian republics which are well within the tourist track, travellers still die of cholera and typhoid each year. Infective hepatitis is not

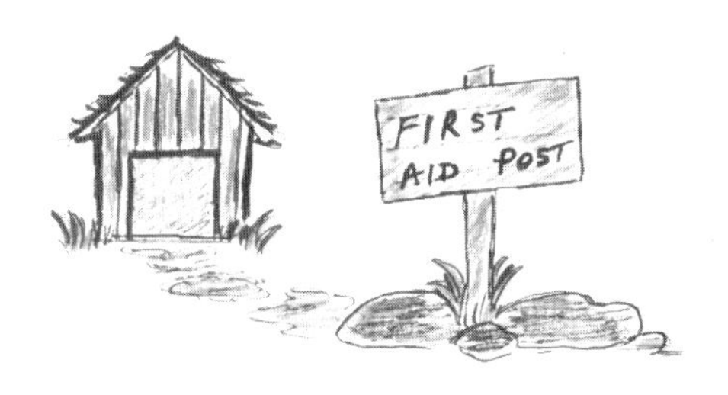

Variable health facilities

just a risk for the back-packer in Nepal. It can affect any tour group with lunchtime stop-overs in underdeveloped countries with low hygiene standards.

Hepatitis B and AIDS transmission prevention packs are now available for purchase from MASTA and have to be a serious consideration for tourists to the up-country areas of Africa and Asia. Patients have also to be advised that, even in Europe reciprocal EC insurance arrangements are rarely adequate to cover them without further expenditure on their part and extra insurance is always advisable.

All foreign travellers should maintain tetanus, tuberculosis and polio protection. Tetanus is always a risk where night-soil is a standard form of crop fertilisation and tuberculosis and poliomylitis are still endemic in many countries. Typhoid vaccination is a standard recommendation but there is dispute over the value of cholera injections for protection is variable. On balance, it is probably still wise to include both in the vaccination programme of a world traveller.

If exposure to diphtheria is likely, for example in India, and there has been no vaccination in the last five years then 'adult' type low dose booster vaccine is adviseable. Back-packers and those going up-country in the Far and Middle East, Russia and Africa are also advised to have gamma globulin if not known to be immune to Hepatitis A. A blood check can be done for Hepatitis A antibody in advance of the injection which is usually required if yellow fever vaccination is indicated.

Yellow fever is a requirement for Africa and South America and is still compulsory for certain countries. It is required for travel to 15 degrees north and 10 degrees south of the Equator in Africa and all parts of South America that are north of 20 degrees south. The vaccination does have the advantage that it lasts for ten years whereas cholera vaccination lasts a mere six months and typhoid vaccination three years.

Advice on appropriate malarial prophylaxis for the travelling patient is best obtained from the nearest local tropical disease unit. It is vital that malaria prophylaxis starts at least one week before exposure to risk and be continued for two weeks after return from the trip. Many patients fail to appreciate the need to continue treatment after their return to the UK.

Drug resistance is an ever increasing problem in much of Africa and a cocktail of drugs is now often required to achieve reasonable protection. Insect bites remain a serious threat abroad and patients should be advised to carry insect repellents and aerosols, and wear sensible protective clothing after dusk. The new rabies vaccine is available for those visiting rural India and South East Asia and requires three injections over five months.

A major element in staying healthy throughout a foreign trip is scrupulous attention to food and water ingestion. Where the latter is concerned, it is wise to always assume contamination and use sterilising tablets or bottled water. Indiscriminate eating of salads and unwashed fruits probably accounts for most attacks of gastroenteritis and it has to be remembered that ice in drinks or ice cream is likely to be contaminated.

Many tourists avoid drinking local water and devour greens and tomatoes on side plates without thought. Cold dishes left exposed to flies are also a high risk and should be avoided.

On holiday in Greece, I once was presented with a four-layered moussaka which on closer inspection had four or five 'blue-bottle' flies incarcerated between each layer. An inspection of the restaurant kitchen revealed swarms of unsavoury insects infesting the food stores.

The Japanese encephalitis vaccine is now being recommended for travellers to endemic areas such as India, Nepal, South East Asia and China where epidemics occur regularly, especially during the rainy season. Three vaccinations are required with a further booster.

Patients are returning from the Carribean with sand-worm infestation of the feet. This infection is rarely considered in diagnosis when seen for the first time in the surgery, but should be kept in mind. Patients should be advised to wear sandals when on the beaches of the Carribean islands.

Family doctors are often asked about appropriate first aid kits for travelling and a few simple remedies can be recommended, such as:

antihistamine tablets and cream
oral rehydrating agents
OTC anti-diarrhoea preparations
wound dressings
adhesive tape
analgesics
water sterilising tablets
antiseptic cream (Savlon)

An important reminder is to ensure that patients take their own personal routine medication with them. Each year patients on long haul flights or lengthy bus trips, go into congestive cardiac failure when they fail to take diuretics.

The Medical Defence Unions have warned that GPs should follow recommended vaccine programmes very closely or face claims for negligence. A recent survey showed only 36% of GPs currently adhered to published advice and were failing to advise and protect their patients adequately. Up-to-date information is now available, in some areas via the Travel Data Base held by the Health Board, or TRAVAX, a computerised travel health information data base available for all GPs with a modem and practice computer (Cossar, 1988), which gives information on vaccination for overseas travel. With sensible preparation, proper vaccination and adequate insurance, the majority of patients can look forward to a healthy holiday.

In the future, many more travellers will undoubtedly venture to increasingly exotic destinations. To travel hopefully and to travel safely is the aim and that requires careful planning, adequate vaccination and an awareness of potential hazards.

References

Cossar J H, Reid D, Fallon R J *et al* (1990). Accumulative review of studies on travellers. *J. Infection*, **21**: 27-42.
Cossar J H, Reid D (1992). Health Advice for Travellers: The Role of the GP, *Health Bulletin* (50) **6**: 428-430.
Cossar J H, Walker E, Reid D, Dewar R D (1988). Computerised advice on malaria prevention and immunisation, *Br Med J*, **296**: 258
D'A Paixo M, Dewar R (1991). What do Scots die of when abroad? *Scot Med J*, **36**: 114-116
Gorman D, Smith B (1992). Travel Agents and Health Advice Given to Holiday Makers, *Trav Med Intnl*, **3**: 111-115
McIntosh I (1991). Travel Induced Illness: A GP-based Survey, *Scot Med*, **11.4**: 14-15.
Reid D, Cossar J (1991). Travel. A health hazard, *Intnl J Environ Health Res*, **1**: 32-36.
Reid D, Cossar J H, Ako T I, Dewar R D (1986). Do travel brochures give adequate advice on avoiding illness, *Br Med J*, **293**: 1472

CHAPTER 1

THE TRAVEL HEALTH CLINIC

The growth of international travel and with it travel-induced illness, has led to an expansion in health promotion services aimed specifically at intending travellers. In a recent British Medical Journal editorial, it was noted that there had been a 23-fold increase in British travellers journeying beyond Europe since the 1950s. In 1990, there were 31 million visits abroad by UK residents (Porter 1992).

Studies in Scotland between 1973 and 1985 showed that 37 percent of travellers developed a related illness (Cossar 1992) and in a published study carried out in my own practice, it was found that no less than 47 percent of travellers aged over 65 years suffered from travel-related illness, 58 percent of these individuals required the attention of their GP on return to the UK and 17 percent required hospital admission (McIntosh 1991).

Despite a wide spectrum of imported disease, there has been a tendency in the past for only malaria and disease preventable by vaccination to receive serious attention from doctors consulted by potential travellers. Advice has often been based only on the geographic situation of the destination.

Travel medicine is becoming a discipline in its own right, recognised by a biennial international conference and the Journal of Travel Medicine International. Health professionals experienced in the field, now recommend that travellers at greatest risk should be identified, the risk quantified and health education targeted towards the nature of the risk and duration of the foreign stay. Spurred on by recent new regulations on health promotion clinics, family doctors are setting up pre-travel health clinics involving counselling, clinical assessment, identification of medical risk and prophylaxis, vaccinations and advice tailored to the individual.

There is a wide range of travel-induced illness. This embraces infection, phobia, motion sickness, jetlag, trauma and disturbances to metabolism, thermal regulation and circadian rhythm. The health counsellor needs to consider the prospective traveller's age, sex, destination and route. The method of travel and exposure to climate, latitude and altitude has to be elicited. Pre-existing illness and appropriate insurance cover are also relevant. There are different risks for the package tourist, the business traveller, the expeditionary, the young, the old, the pregnant, the chronically ill and the disabled.

The travel health clinic

Commercial and gp-organised travel clinics are proliferating worldwide. Doctors and nurses who operate them should be aware of the travel features which have a physical and psychological impact on their clients. Good counselling, appropriate precautions and prophylaxis can diminish the risk of travel-related illness affecting those who journey abroad.

Table 1.1: The effects of travel on the individual

Temperature extremes:-	
High temperature risk	— hyperthermia — heat exhaustion — dehydration
Low temperature risk	— hypothermia — exposure
Humidity	— promotes a disturbance in temperature control
Altitude	— increased risk of acute mountain sickness and hypoxia.
Disturbances in circadian rhythm	— mental change — disturbed metabolism
Air travel	— low partial pressure of oxygen — dry air — contaminated air — jet lag
Sea/land/air transportation	— motion sickness
Cultural shock	— psychological distress
Environmental stress	— noise, delay, re-routing, baggage loss can cause confusion and mental distress
Communication problems	— linguistic and public address system failures and language misunderstanding can cause mental distress
Travel	— the hassle of modern air travel promotes fatigue and psychological disturbance
Physical stress	— long airport walkways, carriage of suitcases, traverse of a maze of stairways and passageways can all be physically demanding
Enforced immobility	— can result in venous thrombosis and pulmonary embolism
Risk of disease	— exotic illness, conditions controlled in the UK, foreign

		infectious disease may result from exposure.
Greater risk of trauma	—	road traffic accident, sports injury, unstable transport medium

Establishing the clinic

This requires good organisation, a sound database, an enthusiastic practice nurse, skilled administration and audit.

A Organising the database

1 Information regarding vaccination schedules can be obtained from Pulse, Doctor or MIMS Magazine Foreign Travel Guides

2 Immunisation against infectious diseases (the Green Book, HMSO 1922)

3 Travel information for medical practitioners (HMSO 1989)

4 Statement of fees and allowances 'Paragraph 27' (the Red Book, HMSO 1992)

5 Advice for travellers (SA 40 HMSO 1992)

6 A Traveller's Guide to Health While You Are Away (SA 41 HMSO 1991)

The latter two publications are information leaflets for patients provided by the government.

7 Travellers Health, Dawood R, Oxford University Press 3rd edn 1992

8 Travel and Health in the Elderly: A medical handbook, McIntosh I, Quay Publishing 1992

B Creation of a management protocol which ought to define objectives, the type of service to be offered, when, by whom and the number of patients likely to be seen during each session.

C Organise administrative details with the practice nurse and the practice manager. Clinic times have to be arranged with appointments at 15 minute intervals. The initial visit is time-consuming but can be shortened by the use of patient questionnaires and a checklist. GP input can be limited to those at high risk and the GP can see patients while the nurse is working in an adjoining room.

D Advertise the clinic in the practice leaflet, the local medical directory and Yellow Pages. Information regarding the clinic can be printed on computerised prescription counterfoils and displayed on the surgery notice boards.

In the past, travel health clinics have been recognised for health promotion payments although regulations are subject to change. Sadly, new rules come into effect April/May 1993 which will exclude travel clinics for health promotion purposes, other than as Well Person Checks

E **Ordering vaccines** – Order vaccines such as tetanus, polio, typhoid, cholera, hepatitis A. Special arrangements may have to be made with the local hospital or laboratory if gamma-immunoglobulin is required. In England, vaccines are often administered by the GPs, saving patients the prescription charge for the costs which can be claimed as personally administered drugs under Section 44 of the Red Book. Any GP south of the Scottish border can dispense vaccines according to Regulation 29/B7b of the terms of service. Scottish GPs are subject to different regulations. Vaccination procedures are not as financially rewarding for Scottish doctors, unless rural practitioners with dispensing status. Most

Scottish doctors obtain vaccines on stock order or by named prescriptions which the patient takes to the local pharmacist. In the latter case, the prescription attracts the Government prescribing charge.

In England, the vaccine should be written as a prescription on FP10 and the FP10s collected until the end of the month when they can be sent to the prescription prescribing authority with a copy of the invoices on FP34D. These can be claimed if done by the practice nurse as she gives the immunisation on the GP's instructions. Immunisations which do not attract a government fee have to be charged against the patient.

F Create a fee schedule

Private fees can be charged for:

a fitness to travel certificate

A non-red book immunisation to NHS patient

Immunisations for private patients

International certificate of vaccination

Freedom from infection report

Holiday cancellation insurance claim certificate

Private prescriptions for medications to be used abroad

Passport counter-signature

After completing the list, it is appropriate to have the patient sign a consent form for vaccination. Despite the legitimate effort to ensure adequate prophylaxis it should be remembered that 95 percent of travel-related disease is not vaccine-preventable. Advice given regarding diet and the treatment of diarrhoea is probably more important than immunisation.

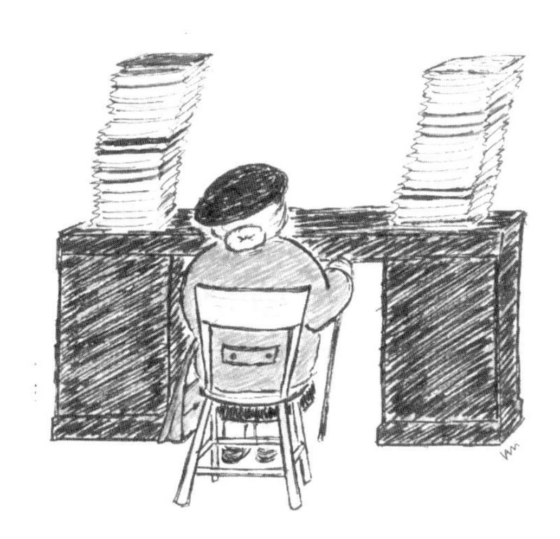

Pre-travel documentation

Verbal advice given at the pre-travel consultation can be reinforced by giving the patient a printed hand-out leaflet.

Appropriate topics for leaflets are:-

Avoiding infected water and contaminated food

Protection against mosquito bites and risks of malarial infection

Skin dangers from exposure to the sun

How to cope with diarrhoeal illness while abroad

(see examples in appendix)

Conflicting advice is given to intending travellers by general practitioners. A Scottish study showed that doctors do not give patients consistent advice on appropriate vaccination (Cossar 1990). This is partly due to a lack of a single information source. The study showed that patients received protection they did not require or was of doubtful value, eg. cholera vaccination was adminstered but protection against polio or tetanus was omitted. Two thirds of travellers departing from the UK reported that they expected to obtain travel advice from their family doctor.

A check-list can be helpful to determine appropriate advice on prophylaxis and, with the use of a standardised health questionnaire for intending travellers, can create an individualised vaccination package.

Patient check-list prior to vaccination

Where is the patient going?

Will the visit be in the dry or wet season, summer or winter?

Is the patient healthy?

Is there a history of chronic illness?

Does the patient have any allergies, eg. to eggs?

Are there contraindications to travel due to current or past disease?

What is the disease prevalence at the destination?

What is the current immune status?

Are there contraindications to prophylaxis in the light of age and possible side-effects?

What are the current medications?

Is the patient taking steroid treatment, cancer therapy, immune suppressive therapy?

Is the patient pregnant?

Immunisations

Schedule of immunisation

Compulsory:	— yellow fever
Commonly recommended	— typhoid fever, hepatitis A, poliomylitis, tetanus
Occasionally recommended	— diptheria, tick-borne encephalitis, cholera and BCG

In practice, two consultations four to six weeks apart, cater for most travellers' needs.

Consultation 1

i) initiate primary course of tetanus toxoid and oral poliomyelitis vaccine if necessary, or boost if no booster within ten years. If the traveller is only going to Europe, USA, Canada, Australia, New Zealand or Japan, no other immunisations are needed.

ii) cholera vaccine can be considered but is very rarely required. It is no longer a WHO recommendation and in the light of its side-effects it should not be given to the old.

iii) give typhoid and hepatitis A vaccines

Consultation 2 (four to six weeks later)

i) confirm that yellow fever vaccination has been given

ii) boost typhoid vaccine with a primary course

iii) give hepatitis A vaccination

Generally no immunisation is required for those travelling to USA, Canada, Northern and Western Europe, Australia and New Zealand where public health standards are high. Travellers to the popular resorts in France, Spain and Italy do not need injections other than tetanus and polio.

Unfortunately, they are at high risk of succumbing to diarrhoeal disease when holidaying along the shores of the Mediterranean Sea. Vacationers to Greece and its islands report a high incidence of travel-related illness. All those visiting the former USSR and eastern bloc countries run a high risk of contracting water- or food-borne disease.

The travel clinic consultation

Assessment and management

A primary objective is to create a customised vaccination programme schedule and health education programme to meed individual needs. The use of a standardised questionnaire does much to provide the necessary information to tailor the response to meet the patient's specific needs.

The questionnaire

This should include a note of:

demographic details, destination, season, method of travel, travel duration, holiday type, climatic hazards, smoking status, functional disability, psychological disturbance, predisposition to travel sickness, previous travel phobias

current physical medical status, pre-existing chronic disease, current mental status

visual acuity, hearing status, vaccination status

potential medical facilities at the destination and insurance cover

Assessing the risk

It is possible to score responses into low, medium and high risk so that those exposed to special risk to their health when abroad can be identified. Patient questionnaires and check-lists are timesaving in identifying risk.

Low risk group

There is usually low risk for those aged 15-65 who are functionally and mentally fit and travelling by air to North America, Northern Europe and the Antipodes, to visit relatives in cities at low altitudes with a good climate

Table 1.1: The low risk group

1.	— those aged 15-65
2.	— the functionally and mentally fit
3.	— those travelling by air to North America, Northern Europe and the Antipodes
4.	— those visiting relatives in cities at low altitudes with a good climate.

High risk group

Very young children, people over 65, travellers to the tropics, South-East Asia, India, the Far East or Africa during the monsoon, are at high risk of suffering travel-related illness. People on safari, up-country adventure, sporting holidays at high altitude or in climatic extremes are also at risk.

Table 1.1: The high risk group

1 — Very young children
2 — people over 65
3 — travellers to the tropics, South East Asia, India, the Far East or Africa during the monsoon
4 — People on safari
5 — up-country adventure holidays
6 — sporting holidays at:
  i) high altitude
  ii) in climatic extremes

The visually impaired, the very deaf and the disabled are also more likely to run into health hazards when travelling.

Table 1.2 The handicapped

1 — the functionally disabled
2 — visually impaired
3 — the very deaf
4 — the disabled

Those who are functionally disabled or suffer from serious cardiovascular, cerebrovascular, renal or hepatic disease, chronic obstructive airways disease or diabetes can put themselves at high risk during long distanced travel.

Table 1.3 Pre-existing illness

those who suffer from:
1 — serious cardiovascular disease
2 — cerebrovascular disease
3 — renal or hepatic disease
4 — chronic obstructive airways disease
5 — diabetes mellitis

Management

Those at low risk may require only general advice and enhanced tetanus protection. Those at medium risk are likely to need a wide range of vaccinations and specialist advice on pre-existing illness and the effects of travel. High risk travellers require a full clinical check and reappraisal of drug requirements with customised advice about travel arrangements.

Everyone who travels to developing countries should be reminded that medical facilities may be inadequate.

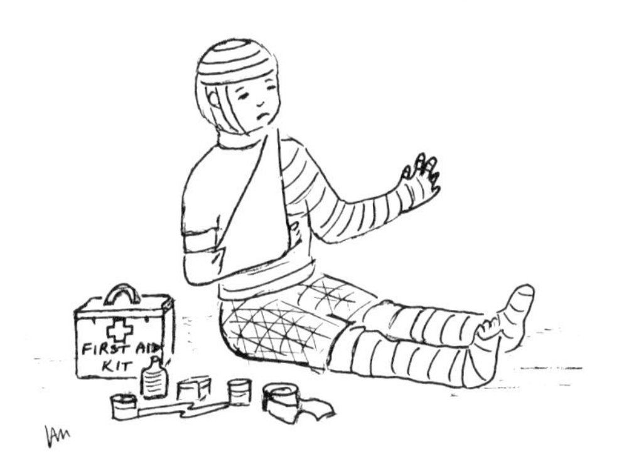

First Aid Measures

Clinics may be devoid of equipment and carry only the simplest of drugs. Sterilisation procedures are often limited, non-disposable syringes may not be available and there may be a high risk of HIV infection or hepatitis transmission. Medical care is likely to be provided by nursing staff constrained by lack of medications, dressings and education.

Hospitals are often over over-crowded, insanitary and equipped with the bare minimum of medical requisites. Patient feeding may depend on that provided by relatives; changing bed linen and attention to toilet needs may only be provided by tipping ward auxillaries. Blood transfusion supplies may not be screened for HIV infection.

Medical aid from a qualified doctor can be hours if not days away. Even when provided, it may be in a form unacceptable to the patient. Suppository and injection medication often supplants tablet medication in eastern parts of Europe and acupuncture, moxibustion and herbal medicine use is common in the Far East.

Emergency transportation

In much of Africa and Asia, ambulances, if available, are often unreliable and unsprung. They may well only turn out or pick up the patient if a fee is paid in advance or if insurance protection is ascertained. In extremis, air evacuation may be logistically impracticable and local aid with all its inadequacies may be the only option.

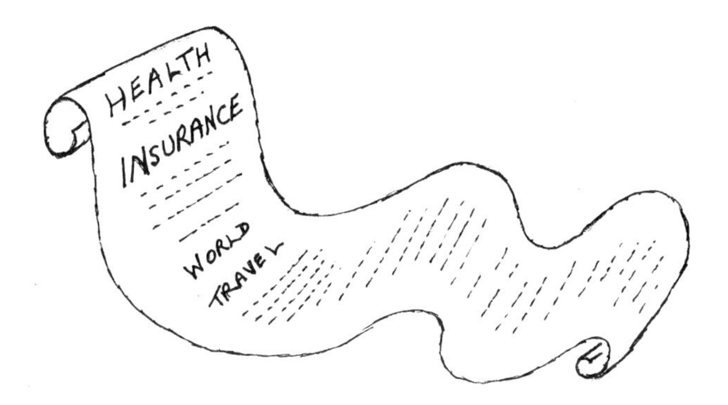

Travel insurance

Adequate travel insurance is a necessity and most pay willingly for medical protection. Expenses covered are, however, often inadequate for visits to the USA. Many people travel without suitable medical insurance protection and even more do so unaware that their insurance excludes pre-existing or recurrent illness. In a study in my practice (N° 745) 62 percent were unaware of the protection they had bought. For a larger premium adequate cover can, invariably, be purchased. Although insurance is a prerequisite, it can only be of value if good local medical facilities are to hand and rapid evacuation to the UK is a practicable possibility. Many travellers venture far afield and into remote parts of the world unaware of its limitations. The travel health counsellor ought to draw attention to this problem and, in the best interests of the less healthy, advise a journey in close proximity to prompt and effective health care.

Practice leaflets

Precautionery advice from the practice nurse and doctor can be reinforced by the use of handouts with written instructions. Typical examples are:

Avoidance of contaminated water

The dangers of infected food

The risk from sunburn and ultraviolet light

Dos and don'ts for safe eating

The hazards of long-haul air flights

Taking travel precautions

(See Appendix)

Large numbers of UK residents travel to European destinations for their holidays, half of them on package tours. As many as 37 percent may be affected by travel-related illness which can spoil the holiday or even be life-threatening. There is a very high incidence of traveller's diarrhoea in those visiting Mediterranean resorts. Protracted vomiting brings a risk of dehydration which can have serious consequences in small children and the elderly.

Strong ultraviolet light plays havoc with the skin and leads not only to the risk of severe sunburn but the possibility of triggering melanoma.

Long-haul air flights put those with chronic obstructive airways disease, myocardial ischaemia and cerebrovascular disease at high risk. Deep venous thrombosis and pulmonary emboli can occur in long-haul air travellers en route to Australia and the Far East. Jet lag can also ruin a holiday or business trip.

Exposure to **high altitude** on visits to Machu Picchu, Mexico, or the Himalayas can cause serious illness and prove fatal. High altitude climbers are at obvious risk but so, too, are many tourists unaware of the altitude to which they are exposed.

All those who venture in and on the water, especially if involved in water sports, are at extra risk from insect bites, coral abrasions and diseases and infestations of the skin.

Risk assessment and management protocols for the travel clinic

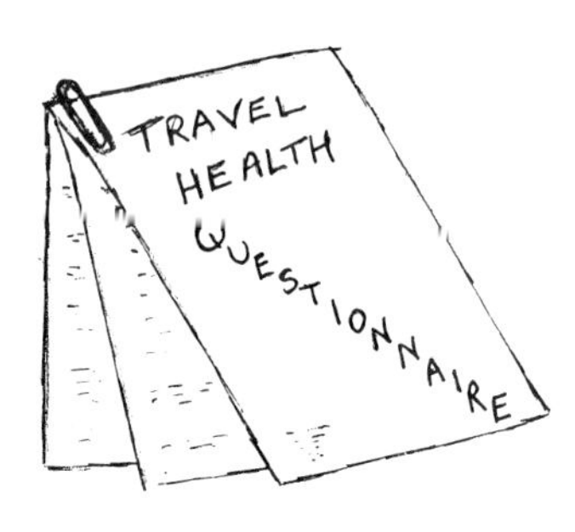

Use of a standard questionnaire will facilitate recognition of higher risk travellers and abbreviated tick-lists can be self-adminstered to save time.

Those suffering from pre-existing disease are less able to compensate for the demands of a hostile environment and are more likely to succumb to travel-induced illness and disease. After completion, the questionnaire can be scored for risk by nurse or doctor.

A standardised questionnaire

Tick√	Demographic Details	Risk (circle)		
		Low	Med	High
	Age			
	65–78	*		
	75–85		*	
	85+			*
	Destination			
	North Europe/Canada/America/ New Zealand/Australia	*		
	Eastern Europe/The Eastern Block/ Mediterranean Littoral		*	
	Tropics/South East Asia/India/Far East/Africa			*
	Season			
	Favourable	*		
	Inclement/monsoon		*	
	Transport mode			
	Air		*	
	Sea	*		
	Land	*		
	Travel duration			
	Short	*		
	Long-haul		*	
	Holiday type			
	Visit to relatives/city tours	*		
	Safari/Up-Country/Adventure/ Sporting			*
	Climatic hazard			
	Moderate climate/low altitude	*		
	Climatic extremes/high altitude			*
	Smoking status			
	Non-smoker	*		
	Smoker		*	

Questionnaire (contd)

Tick√	Demographic Details	Risk (circle)		
		Low	Med	High
	Functional disability			
	None	*		
	Pre-existing functional defect		*	
	Incontinence		*	
	Psychological disturbance			
	Stable personality	*		
	Phobia/confusional state/anxiety		*	
	Predisposition to motion sickness			
	Absent	*		
	Definite		*	
	Current physical status			
	Healthy	*		
	Moderately healthy		*	
	Poor health			*
	Pregnancy status			
	Non-pregnant	*		
	Pregnant			*
	Pre-existing Chronic Disease			
	Renal and hepatic disease		*	
	Cardiovascular/cerebrovascular disease		*	
	Diabetes mellitis			*
	Chronic obstructive airways disease			*
	Current mental status			
	Normal	*		
	Disturbed/diminished			*
	Visual acuity			
	Normal	*		
	Diminished		*	
	Vaccination status			
	Full protection	*		
	Absent. No previous vaccinations			*
	Special considerations			
	Terminal illness			*
	Potential medical facilities			
	North Europe/New Zealand/ Australia/North America	*		
	Africa/Asia		*	
	Up-Country/remote destinations			*

Questionnaire (contd)

Tick√	Demographic Details	Risk (circle)		
		Low	Med	High
	Insurance			
	Adequate	*		
	Exclusion clauses		*	
	Absent insurance			*

Management plan

Creation of a customised management plan to minimise risk of potential travel for the individual is recommended.

1 Evaluate the risk using the type of questionnaire suggested

2 Advise the patients of their current risk status with the proposed travel itinerary

3 Identify factors which can be altered to decrease the risk

4 Provide adequate prophylaxis and vaccination

5 Provide appropriate advice regarding precautions to be taken en route and at the destination and for considerations promoting extra risk

6 Counsel on appropriate changes in drug medication, e.g. with a diabetic or dietary change and how to deal with alterations in circadian rhythm

7 Advise regarding minimising the effects of pre-existing disease during travel and on holiday

8 Provision of appropriate certificates and referral letters and completion of any certificates required by transport authorities or tour operators.

9 Advise patients of sources of information booklets etc which may find of value

A clinical valuation will be required for the very frail old or for those with pre-existing disease. This may exclude from travel or may require special considerations in travel. Much of the assessment in the above procedures can be carried out by other members of the Primary Care Team, such as the nursing sister or other attached health professionals. The whole procedure can be undertaken as part of a health promotion clinic or as part of the contractual assessment for the over 75 year old patient.

Minimising the risks of route and venue

Destination

It may be quite inappropriate for the patient to visit the proposed destination, eg those with chronic obstructive airways disease wanting to visit places at high altitude. Alternatives may be acceptable in the pre-planning stage.

Season

It is wise for the patients to travel when climatic extremes are least hazardous.

Transport mode

For some patients air transportation may be unacceptable although there are few exclusions. Shorter flights or transit stops may be advisable and sea travel in calm seas is, perhaps, the safest mode of transportation for the old. Sea cruises are a low risk form of travel, invariably with good medical facilities as a back-up.

Holiday type

Patients at risk may need to be dissuaded from undertaking cultural visits to the Valley of the Kings where ambient temperatures lie well above 100 degrees fahrenheit or to Inca sights in South America at high altitude. The popular safari trips round Africa may also offer unacceptable hazards to the individual.

The functionally disabled

This group is well catered for with special support available at many international airports and destinations but facilities may be grossly inadequate or non-existent in developing countries during transit or stop-over.

Psychological disturbances

Travel phobias (Chapter 4) respond well to treatment and with pre-planning a course of desensitisation will be able to free the passsenger from this problem.

Motion sickness

The prescription of any pill will bring a high positive placebo response but scopaderm patches and other anti-emetic tablets can diminish this problem (see Chapter 5).

Pre-disposing illness

These patients require additional counselling.

Drugs

The diabetic and the asthmatic are particularly at risk and changes in circardian rhythm require changes in times of medication with these groups.

Medical facilities

These are very variable internationally, a feature of which many travellers are unaware having been protected by the National Health Service for most of their lifetime.

Insurance

It is absolutely vital that individuals leave the country with adequate insurance for every eventuality. It must also be remembered that the protection provided by insurance is only as good as the facilities on the ground at the chosen destination and that air evacuation may well take days to organise in some of the more remote places of the world.

References

Cossar J A (1990). A cumulative review of studies of travellers. *J Infect*, **21**, 27–42.
McIntosh I (1991). Travel-induced illness - a GP based survey. *Scot Med*, **11**, 4, 14–5.
Porter J D (1992). Editorial, *B M J*, **304**, 1324–5.

CHAPTER 2

POOR HYGIENE AND DISEASE

A common observation is that travel may broaden the mind but it will also loosen the bowels and about a third of international travellers will suffer bowel disorder whilst abroad. At best, an inconvenience, it may mean missed business or holiday opportunities, debilitation and in the very young or old it can be life threatening.

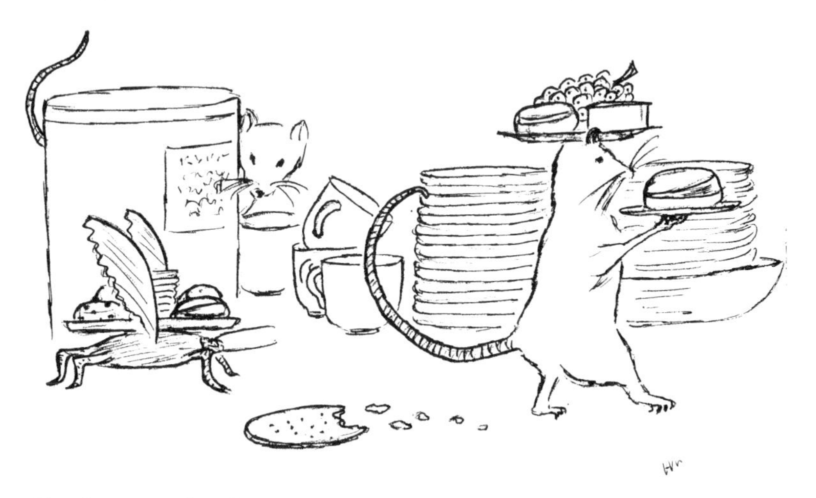

Food contamination

Travellers' diarrhoea is the single most common health problem for travellers, with bacterial agents accountable for 80 percent of the cases. The back-packer, those living in rural communities in the developing world, the old and very young are at extra risk. The old often develop auto immune deficiencies that may predispose them to infectious diarrhoea. Decreased host immunity correlates with increasing age and the risk of serious bloodstream *Salmonella* infection is increased in the elderly. Diabetic neuropathy, anticholinergics, H_2 blockers and antacids also alter intestinal clearance of bacteria.

Scrupulous attention to food and water hygiene offers the traveller the best chance of avoiding the scourge. If foodstuffs cannot be boiled, cooked or peeled they are best left alone on foreign travel. Recent reports suggest a reduction in duration and intensity of the disorder by 50 percent with treatment using bismuth subsalicylate. Loperamide gives an 80 percent decrease of diarrhoea in apyrexial patients free from dysentery. The treatment for moderate to severe diarrhoea and dysentery is trimethoprim/ sulfmethoxazole or a quinolone for areas where antimicrobial resistance is a problem.

Responsible organisms are:

E.Coli	40%
Shigella	15%
Salmonellas	10%
Rotaviruses	10%
Giardia lamblia	3%
Entamoeba histolytica	3%
Enteropathogens	cholera and typhoid

Viral hepatitis

Hepatitis A (HAV) infection

There are two main kinds of viral hepatitis, one being hepatitis A which is also referred to as infectious hepatitis and the other hepatitis B. Hepatitis A occurs endemically in many parts of the world especially where there is overcrowding, poor hygiene with inadequate water supplies and lack of sanitation. Travellers to areas outwith industrialised Europe, North America, Australia and New Zealand can become infected and succumb to an unpleasant disease often of prolonged duration. Several different viruses are implicated and vaccination has become available to combat the impact of hepatitis A and B. (Figure 2.3).

The virus causes an acute inflammation of the liver with symptoms of fever, chill, fatigue, weakness, aches and pains and headache. Later, nausea, vomiting and anorexia, upper abdominal pain, jaundice, pigmented urine and light coloured stools can occur. In the young many infections are symptomless but jaundice can be severe and the illness prolonged, with even liver failure and ensuing coma. Although there is a low associated mortality, sufferers may be incapacitated for months and a mortality of 1.5 percent in people aged over 64 years, has been recorded by the UK Public Health Laboratory Service for those with fulminant hepatitis A infection. Data from the United States Department of Health and Human Services indicates that mortality rate may be up to 2.7 percent in those over 40 years of age. Underlying liver disease may have been a factor in some of these cases. The viral incubation period is 35 weeks, with faecal shedding and infectivity greatest during this time. As many as 10 percent of hepatitis A patients are estimated to relapse (Gocke, 1986).

In 1990 there were 7,316 notifications of hepatitis A in England and Wales, and 435 for hepatitis B. Data presented at a recent international symposium held in Vienna, suggested that 30 million travellers from industrialised countries visit endemic areas annually. Perhaps as many as 40 percent of cases of hepatitis A are associated with recent international travel. HAV is, therefore, a major source of morbidity in travellers to developing countries, with an estimated incidence among unprotected travellers as high as 20 per 1000 for each month of stay in an endemic area. The exact incidence is difficult to determine due to the occurrence of a high proportion of asymptomatic cases. HAV is often contracted by those travelling from areas of low to high prevalence, with all age groups susceptible. An Italian study has shown that the risk of contracting the disease varies with the destination.

Risk of contracting Hepatitis A

1.0	the non traveller,
2.6	travellers to Southern Italy
5.9	visitors to Eastern Europe and the Mediterranean
25.2	travellers to Africa, Asia, Southern and Central America.

The risk is also correlated with the mode of travel, highest risk being among backpackers and travellers staying in primitive and rural conditions.

In non-industrialised and developing countries, HAV infection is usually acquired sub clinically in childhood but with improving standards of hygiene, children escape infection until infected clinically in young adulthood. It is spread from person to person by faecal/oral transmission resulting from faecal contamination of food and water. Food-borne outbreaks are becoming more common in developed countries. Raw vegetables, fertilised with human night soil, and raw or poorly cooked shellfish grown in polluted waters, are recognised as highly infective sources of HAV.

The wise traveller can take some preventive measures by avoiding ingestion of uncooked shell-fish and raw vegetables, and drinking only sterilised water and milk. The injection of human normal immunoglobulin (HNIG) consists of antibodies derived from pooled human serum. In recent years it has been used to promote short-term protection, but the injection was often painful and this passive immunisation gives protection which lasts for only a few months. As antibody levels decline from the time of the injection, frequent travellers have to endure repeated injections. A further disadvantage is that immunoglobulin cannot be administered at the same time as, or, in close time proximity to, other live vaccines such as poliomyelitis.

Hepatitis A virus was propagated in tissue culture in 1979 and a new inactivated vaccine, Havrix, has recently been licensed in the UK. The vaccine is well tolerated and highly immunogenic.

The level and quality of the immune response achieved by a vaccine is important. In studies involving over 1000 healthy volunteers one month after vaccination with an initial dose of **Havrix®**, 95.6 percent of the trial subjects had seroconverted.

The geometric mean anti-HAV titres were approximately ten times higher than those occurring after a passive immunisation. This response is more than sufficient to protect against hepatitis A infection. After a second dose of **Havrix®** one month later, the seroconversion rose to 99.9 percent and the anti-HAV titres rose by about two thirds. **Havrix®** is a major advance in HAV protection, comparing favourable with passive immunity from immunoglobulin injection. The latter is a plasma product which is safe and efficacious, and relatively inexpensive but it gives only short-term protection for about five months, and its protection may decline with falling levels of immunity in developed countries. Three doses of **Havrix®** will produce antibody concentrations over 100 times higher than HNIG injection and are expected to provide immunity for up to ten years.

It is cost effective to use **Havrix®** for vaccination of regular international travellers to areas with poor standards of food and water hygiene. The consensus opinion, at the second Conference of International Association of Travel Medicine in 1991, encouraged hepatitis vaccination of all susceptible travellers to such areas from low endemicity regions such as the UK. In Britain the DHS recommends that travellers to all countries outside Northern or Western Europe, Northern America, New Zealand and Australia should be protected against hepatitis A infection. There is a case for selective blood screening for antibodies before giving a vaccination to older European and American adults who may already be immune.

Visitors to Africa, Asia and South and Central America who are likely to be 'living rough' or to areas of primitive sanitation and contaminated water supplies should certainly receive the vaccine.

Hepatitis B (HBV)

This infection also occurs world-wide, with an estimated 1 in 2500 travellers developing symptoms after returning home. The virus is spread by carriers, or from the infected, during the incubation period or illness. Prevalence varies markedly across the world, with 5 percent of the population carriers in Central and Eastern Europe and 20 percent in parts of Africa, Asia and the Pacific.

The incidence is highest in adults living in squalor in urban and rural areas. Transmission is by skin penetration and infectivity is related to blood, usually resulting from accidental inoculation or by procedures using inadequately sterilised needles and syringes. HBV surface antigen has been found in saliva, menstrual, vaginal and seminal fluid and is probably also transmitted by sexual contact.

World travellers are frequently involved in road traffic accidents, with the possibility of admission to hospitals and clinics where sterilisation procedures may be suspect. There is also a high risk of HBV transmission in the developing countries of Asia and Africa. Homosexual and drug-abusing travellers expose themselves to the risk of infection, and tattooing, chiropody, dentistry and intrusive medical attention where there has been inadequate sterilisation of instruments, place the tourist at risk. Mechanical transmission by biting insects such as bed-bugs and mosquitoes may also occasionally spread the disease.

The world traveller should avoid penetration of the skin by objects previously in contact with the blood of others. Razor and needle-sharing should be eschewed and acupuncture, chiropody and dental treatment is best left until the return home. The possibility of infection must be kept in mind if over zealous border officials insist on pre-entry cholera vaccination where syringes and needles may possibly be contaminated.

Active immunisation with hepatitis B vaccine is practicable if relatively expensive and should be considered for long-stay travellers to endemic areas and 'at risk' groups working in tropical and sub-tropical areas.

Human immunodeficiency virus (HIV)

HIV is a world wide problem with choice of destination less important than the behavioural pattern of the traveller on business, tour or holiday. The World Health Organisation has estimated that ten million adults are infected across the world, with a million infected in the USA. Sexual and drug-using behaviour rather than the geographic location usually determine the risk to the traveller. However, in poor and developing countries, in rural areas and up-country where disposable medical equipment is not available, the re-use of needles and

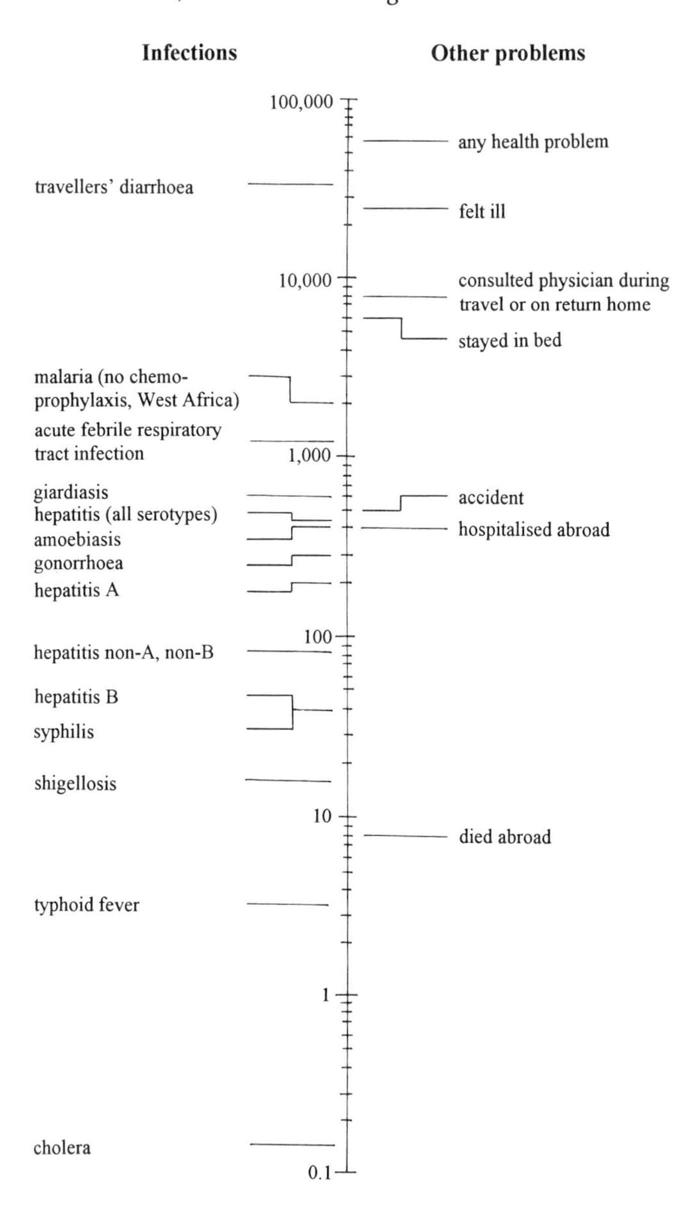

Figure 2.3: Monthly incidence of health problems per 100,000 travellers to tropical areas: *R. Steffen, Proceedings of 2nd Internat. conference on Travel Medicine, Atlanta 1991*

syringes permits blood contamination of instruments and is a potential source of infection to the unwary recipient.

Road traffic accidents are common hazards abroad, and emergency admission to hospitals and clinics in some countries in Africa and Asia have the added risk of transfusion with blood or blood products, where blood donations from the local population have been inadequately screened or treated.

Travellers engaging in sexual and drug-taking behaviour are at high risk if in contact with people who might be HIV infected. If indulging in these activities when abroad, they should be encouraged to use safe sexual practices and condoms. If re-use of medical equipment is common in the country being visited, it is vital to ensure that medical carers are trained in good sterilisation and infection control procedures. Outwith Western Europe, North America, Japan, Australia and New Zealand, adequate screening of donated blood is the exception rather than the rule. WHO now believes that most capital cities have at least one source of screened blood for transfusion. The risks of blood transfusion with infected blood are, therefore, high in many parts of the world and must be taken into consideration by the world traveller. Dental, chiropody and acupuncture treatment is better left until the return home and tourists are well-advised to travel with a well equipped first aid kit, complete with a few disposable syringes and needles.

HIV disease will continue to attract international attention and travel-related HIV infection has to be considered when counselling the traveller. Injecting drug abusers and the sexually promiscuous are most at risk. For the majority of global travellers, travelling to countries of high or intermediate HAV endemicity there is a much greater likelihood of them succumbing to hepatitis HAV infection. Steffen has estimated that susceptible travellers have a risk of 3-6 hepatitis A infections per 1000 months of

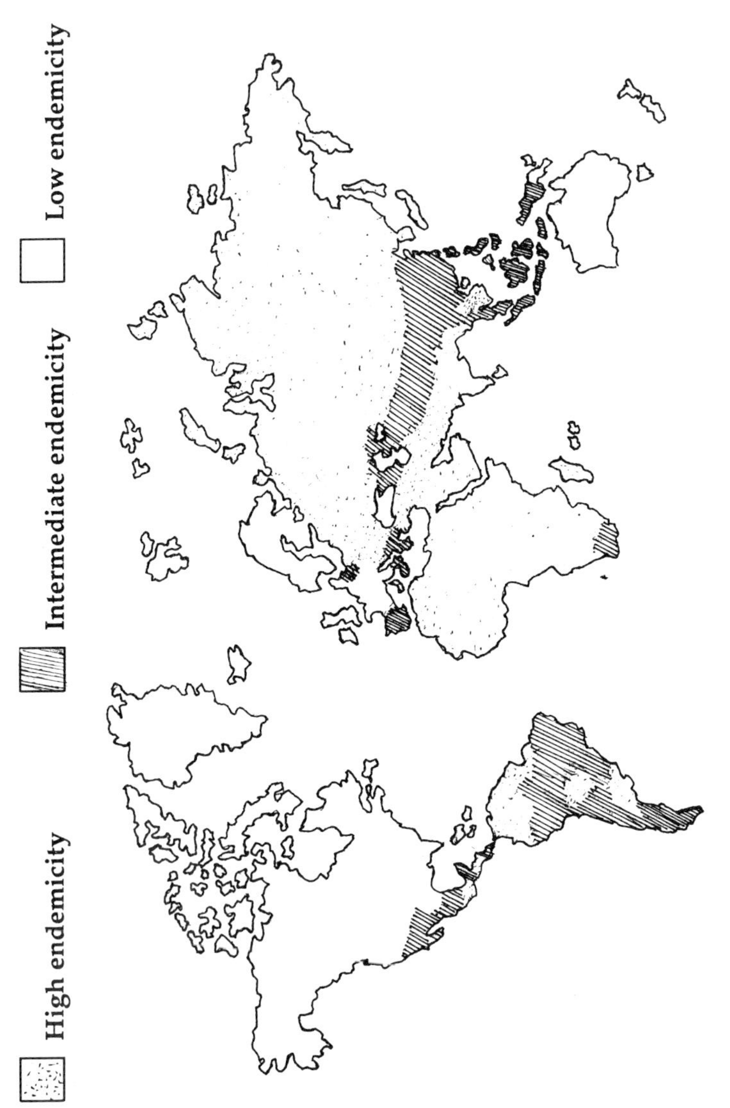

Figure 2.3 Hepatitis A - World Epidemiology

travel in less developed countries and for off-beat travellers this risk may be six times higher. Little as yet can be done for those suffering from HIV infection but vaccination can now protect the majority of international tourists and backpackers from travel-induced hepatitis.

Ringing the changes in travel vaccination

Cholera

Mandatory cholera vaccination was introduced by WHO in 1969 and after its failure to prevent the cross-border spread of the disease was abandoned in 1973. The ultimate ending of routine recommendation of the vaccine for travellers ought to have come with the demise of cholera vaccination certification in 1989. However, one million pounds are still spent annually in the UK on the product. The vaccine can produce a false sense of security for it only protects about 50 percent of those injected who are exposed to the disease. Some patients are encouraged to have the injection by the fear that border officials may insist on vaccination at the border crossing, with the risk of Hepatitis and HIV transmission from poorly sterilised equipment. Scrupulous food and water hygiene precautions will protect most travellers. Despite the recent outbreak in South America, WHO is not currently recommending the use of the cholera vaccine.

Typhoid

There are now two possible routes for administering typhoid vaccine oral and injectable. The former **vivotif®** is a live vaccine, oral strain Ty 21a which comes in a blister pack as a course of three capsules to be swallowed on alternate days. The product has been available in parts of Europe, USA and Australia for some years. It gives protection within 712 days and lasts for three years. There is a very low incidence of mild gastro intestinal side-effects and it should not be given concomitantly with antibiotics or merloquine. More expensive than parenteral protection, its needle-free administration will undoubtedly make it popular with patients once its existence becomes widely known.

Conventional two dose injectable vaccine has always been associated with local pain and swelling at the injection site, pyrexia and headache. A new one shot injectable typhime Vi with apparently fewer local reactions and perhaps three percent systemic reactions is now prescribable.

Hepatitis A

The new vaccine against hepatitis A infection - **Havrix®** - is now available with three injectable doses necessary for long-term protection. Dearer than gamma globulin but less painful for the recipient, it offers protection over several years and will be welcomed by frequent travellers who have endured repeated gamma globulin injections. A blood test can check immunity to hepatitis A before giving the vaccine and its administration is particularly important for backpackers and those visiting rural areas in developing or third world countries.

References

Gocke D J (1986). Hepatitis A Revisited (Editorial), *Ann Intl Med*, **105**, 960

Hadler S (1990). *Global Impact of Hepatitis A Virus Infection Changing Patterns*, International Symposium on Viral Hepatitis and Liver Disease, Houston, Texas (Proceedings)

Steffen R (1991). The Epidemiologic Basis for the Practice of Travel Medicine, 10-15, Travel Medicine 2, Inter Socy Trav Med.

US Department of Health and Human Services (1987). *Hepatitis Surveillance (CDC)*, **51**, 18.

CHAPTER 3

THE STRESS OF MODERN TRAVEL

Summary

Travel by road, rail and air for business or leisure is now a prominent feature of everyday living. The risks to life and limb of different modes of transport used in relocation are quantifiable. Hazards can be identified and countered by the individual and the state. The psychological trauma of global transit is not so well appreciated and documented. Many people are unprepared for the stress engendered by national and international travel.

Relocation is itself a stressor and routine stress tests recognise the significant effect on the individual of a recent foreign holiday (Lucas 1987).

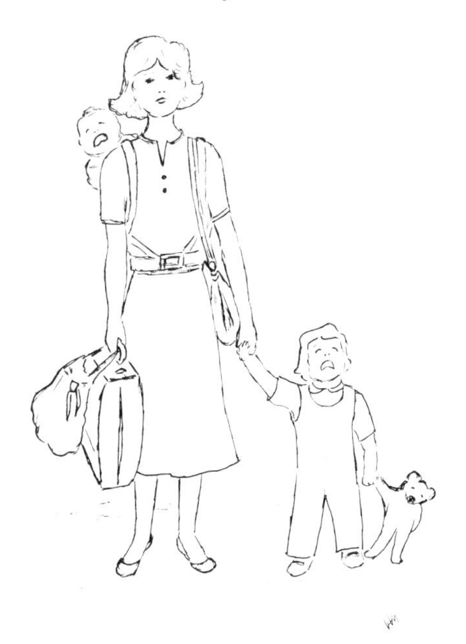

Figure 3.1: Travel and Stress

As in many disease processes, the elderly may suffer disporportionately (McIntosh 1991). Longer flights and faster road speeds with congested air and roadways have made road and air travel more stressful.

Air Travel

Pre-flight anxieties

En route delays on crowded motorways ensure that many travellers are under stress by the time they reach their point of departure, in the endeavour to meet temporal deadlines imposed by airlines and travel companies. Commercial travel fosters anxiety with its endless possibilities for missed flights, lost luggage, cross-border and customs inquisitions, and transportation delays.

Gone are the days when one could enter the airport, purchase a ticket, dispose of luggage, stroll out to the aircraft and anticipate prompt departure. Now, security demands dictate a one to two hour pre-flight routine, involving passenger segregation, security screening, the intrusion of body searches and emigration control. Added to inevitable strikes by handlers, air-crew and air traffic controllers, lengthy delays are the distressing norm for intercontinental air journeys. The individual is exposed to considerable environmental stress at a time of maximal vulnerability (Pollit 1986).

Air travellers may be close to their stress tolerance threshold before they even leave the passenger concourse to brave the perceived hazards of the actual flight. On long-delayed departures, even apparently psychologically-stable married couples may develop acute inter-personal tension, dependent upon their coping abilities and reactions, in response to the uncontrolled situation in which they find themselves.

Stressors

Apprehension is initially generated by pre-flight security, baggage and personal searches which although prudent, are a reminder of the risk of hijack and in-flight explosion. The surrender of baggage brings legitimate worries about its mis-routing or total loss. Inaudible communications, poor acoustics, incomprehensible visual displays, overcrowding and a surfeit of noise can disturb and disorientate the seasoned traveller, provoke anxiety in the novice and seriously confuse the elderly and mentally unstable.

Table 3.1 Air travel stressors

Air travel stressors
Protracted ticket procedures
Security searches
Baggage loss
Overcrowded lounges
Flight delays
Re-routing
Inaudible communications
Inadequate visual displays
Fear of flying

On the air-side of the airport, passengers are at the mercy of an impersonal system reducing the status of the individual to a flight and seat number. There is total dependence upon the unseen whim of airport, airline and air traffic authorities. The unpredictable element in actual flight departure adds to psychological pressures and is aggravated further when delay occurs after loading and passengers are incarcerated in the aircraft on the airfield. The invariable lack of accurate information regarding the cause and probable length of the hold-up compounds passengers' unease.

The impact of these pre-flight stressors and inticipation of a stressful flight encourage passengers to seek relief of anxiety from the airport bar. Ideally, alcohol ingestion should be avoided before and on long air trips as it promotes dehydration. It also potentiates the tranquillisers and hypnotics that many travellers use on their air voyages.

The former are used as anxiolytics and antiphobics. Flying phobia is common and passage through a congested departure hall may test the agoraphobic beyond endurance. Setting foot in the narrow confines of an aeroplane brings panic to the claustrophobic whilst closing of the aircraft doors heightens phobic anxiety in others (McIntosh 1989). Once airborne, fear of flying unsupported in space will bring others close to hysteria (see Chapter 4 on phobias). Hyperventilation is the most frequently encountered cause of distress during commercial air travel.

Case History 3.1

One of my patients, a businessman, forced into air travel by his job, hastens to his allotted place, clamps on the belt, grabs the seat arms, closes his eyes and sweats his way through the flight refusing to leave his refuge until safely on the ground again.

Transmeridian disturbance

Transmeridian flights cause desynchronisation of circadian rhythm. Adjustment may take up to 14 days and mental performance is poorest at the time corresponding to night on the old and new local times. Time-zone changes can be related to affective illness. In a study of patients admitted from Heathrow airport to a psychiatric unit (Jauhar and Weller 1982), depression occurred significantly more often on flights from east to west and hypomania was inversely related to depression in east to west comparison. Rapid time-zone changes appear to precipitate affective illness in the predisposed. Disturbances in circadian rhythms have been previously noted in affective illness. Sleep deprivation and phase advance of the sleep cycle have been used to treat depression and narcosis to treat hypomania. It is not therefore surprising, that there is an association with depressive illness in east to west travel where there is phase retardation in the sleep-wake cycle.

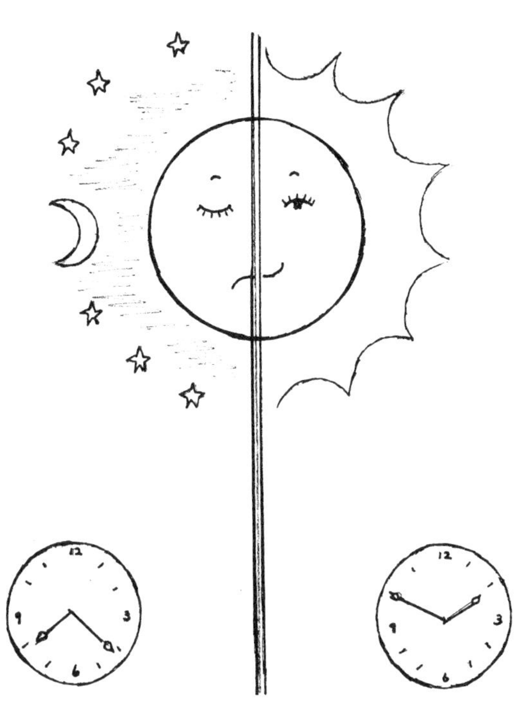

Figure 3.2: Change in Circadian Rhythm

The mentally unstable

Misguided advice to have a break, take a holiday and get away from it all, exposes the undiagnosed depressed patient unnecessarily to the hazards of travel. Disillusioned, depressed patients cannot cope with rapid transit and environmental change, and their condition will deteriorate further. They should be positively discouraged from undertaking relocation until well again. In hypomania and mania, travelling and keeping on the move is often the first overt sign of mental disturbance and forewarns of the potential onset of euphoria and elation. These patients create their own travel difficulties in confrontation with fellow travellers and the authorities. Some voyagers on long round-the-world trips, or intending migrants, find difficulty in adjusting to strange countries and new cultures, and may develop a feeling of paranoia in the first month or two abroad. The cultural shock of visits to Asia and Africa can be intensely disturbing; poverty, racism, religious extremism and bureaucracy can produce alienation and hostility in the travel novice. Many react by isolating and insulating themselves from the local populace in the safety of tour groups and international hotels.

Jet lag

Daily rhythms occur with all physiological, biochemical and psychological variables. Circadian rhythms are caused by complex interaction of 'body clock' habits and external environment. The bio clock is a poor time-keeper but it is adjusted by zeitbergers to the solar day. It provides information about time zone transition. Zeitbergers include rhythms of bright light, sleep, physical activity and social factors. Jet lag is the lack of adjustment between the body clock and local time with speedy crossing of several time-zones). Adjustment to westward travel is easier than that to the east because the body clock tends to run slow and can be delayed more easily than it can be advanced.

Symptoms:
poor sleep
fatigue
headache
disorientation
poor concentration

loss of appetite
made worse with:
increasing number of time zones crossed
increasing age of traveller
eastward rather than westward flights.

Fears and phobias

Fear of black people or of the natives cocoons many a first-time traveller in the tour coach, the tourist-trap, the night-club and on the 'whites only' beach. These fears are sometimes fostered by state agencies short on policing facilities and tour operators intent on maximising profits. They propagate stories of theft and assault on city streets and resort beaches to herd naive tourists towards in-house commercial entertainment.

Foreign travel is often a journey into the unknown and a challenge for some. For others it is a fearsome undertaking. Cruises attract the lonely and depressed seeking company and change (Pollitt 1986). Studies have shown that unpleasant circumstances increase the individual's desire to be with others – 'misery loves company'.

Inherent psychological dangers in group travel

Protected by the agency, the tour guide and the programme, travellers are packaged around the tourist world. Unwittingly enveloped in group psychology they unthinkingly accept the rules of the group, adhere to schedules, join in events; as cogs in a wheel they become part of a gregarious whole. There are, however, inherent psychological dangers for those who will not or cannot participate as they can be ostracised and excluded from the social interaction. The reticent, the retiring, the introverted and the depressed may find themselve unwittingly in, but not belonging to, the group they have joined for security. Actively belonging to a cohesive functioning group can make or mar the holiday. People are inclined to affiliate with others when apprehensive about forthcoming events (Davis 1969). The tourist masses minimise their fears by immersing themselves in group travel and journey, lemming-like, across the continents.

Loneliness of the solo traveller

Swept to the fringe of a group, an individual may be exposed to the loneliness which can engulf the solo adventurer. Some travel to be alone but many seek the solace of the crowd, and a congested airport concourse, a packed '747' or a foreign city street can be a lonely intimidating place for the solo traveller. Home-sickness and feelings of solitude and being unwanted can overtake the international business tycoon, the jet-setter and those on a holiday break. The anonymity of another stereotyped hotel room and the prospect of a solitary evening ahead, push many businessmen towards the hotel bar and an over-indulgence in alcohol.

Sudden environmental change, rapid transit, upset circadian rhythm, hypoxia and anxiety can precipitate the elderly into a state of mental confusion and this group is particularly at risk in long distance travel. Even the young can display confusion when suddenly disembarked at airports situated at high altitude. Anoxia can mentally disturb visitors on the Inca trail to Machu Picchu in Peru or on the Annapurna trekking circuit in Nepal.

Transmeridian flight causes sleep disturbance and the upset in the sleep-wake cycle can bring sleep deprivation with irritability, confusion and personality change. Polar exploration has been related to personality alteration due to the effects of change in the duration of daylight. 'Arctic hysteria' and sleep deprivation occur in those exposed to prolonged daylight and visitors to the Arctic in winter are often overtaken by morbid depression in response to long hours of darkness.

Road travel

Convential road travel in developing countries can be a frightening experience with unskilled drivers driving too fast, in unsafe vehicles, on narrow roads traversed by wandering peasants and slow-moving bullock carts. Even the hardened traveller will become apprehensive when it becomes obvious that the driver is high on drugs.

Case history 3.1

I had a terrifying experience on a coach journey from Cappodocia to Istanbul when the Turkish driver repeatedly endeavoured to steer the bus with his feet and violently resisted efforts to remove him from the driving seat. Women passengers on a tour bus in Nicaragua were reduced to hysteria by the performance of a drunken driver who ultimately bounced the vehicle off a bridge

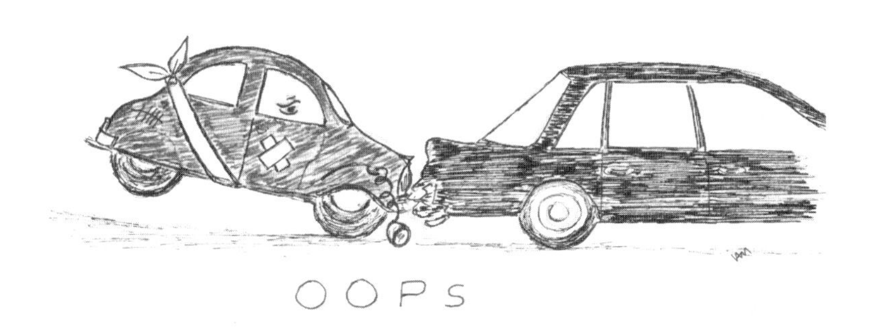

Hazards of land travel

and into a gully. Teenage drivers in Bhutan, which has only recently seen the advent of the motor car, competively race tour cars with death defying bravado on spiralling single-track roads fringed by vertical drops of thousands of feet. Tourists on the Great Trunk Road through India dice with death as drug-besotted and somnambulant truck drivers weave through the traffic. The most sanguine of travellers is likely to become stressed and phobic when exposed to such aberrant road behaviour.

International travel and foreign visits can, therefore, prove to be sources of stress as well as relaxation. They can provide a rich experience, be tedious and boring or act as potent stressors. Recognition of the stresses inherent in travel, sensible anticipation and preparation for potential problems can, however, minimise the pressures and alleviate the strains of global voyaging.

Management

Counter measures

1. Pre-travel seat booking diminishes hassle. Early airport arrival eases time constraints and eliminates the risk of being 'dumped' on over-booked flights.

2. A low-profile through security checks and absence of electronic and electric personal effects in the baggage, decreases the risk of anxiety-provoking, intensive security screening. The phobic can be offered behaviour therapy or hypnotherapy. A graduated treatment programme can be initiated 1 or 2 months before departure. See chapter 4.

3. Alcohol avoidance is recommended on long haul flights but a high fluid intake on the flight and in hot countries is vital as mental performance falls off with even mild dehydration.

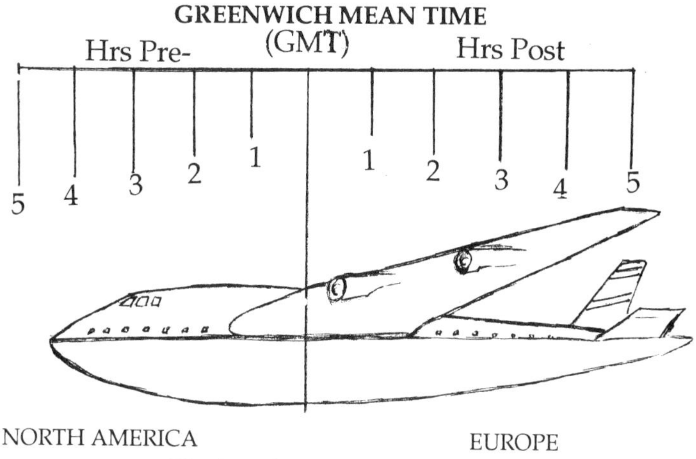

Figure 3.3: Jet-lag

4. There is a case for a mild hypnotic to diminish sleep disturbance in transmeridian journeys and assist sleep at unusual times in the conventional sleep cycle. Benzodiazepines have been shown to facilitate time shifts and if only used for a night or two are unlikely to result in dependence. Time zone adjustment can be promoted by immediate involvement in new time zone routines, eg. for meals and sleep. Adaptation is slower in eastward flights and the middle-aged and elderly seem most affected. One day per hour time-change is needed for the body to 'catch up' with time-changes. Business men should allow three days to elapse before important decision-making meetings after long transmeridian flights. It is best to arrive at the final destination in the evening and take advantage thereafter of midday naps. Rigorously adopt the local time and use zeitgebers at appropriate times to speed up adjustment to new times. (Waterhouse 1992). Mental disturbance is most pronounced at times corresponding to night time on the 'old' and the 'new' local times.

Family doctors should be prepared to counsel their world-travelling patients on the psychological aspects of global relocation (Calder and Wilder 1989), keeping in mind that the elderly and the anxiety-prone are most likely to suffer actual mental trauma. They should be aware of the psychological contraindications to changes in environment for the depressed and the manic, and appreciate how trans-world flying and touring can prove to be a cause of anxiety. From planning to arrival, international journeys and foreign holidays should provide stimulation, satisfaction and enjoyment. An awareness of transit stressors and the adoption of coping strategies can counter the stress which is the inevitable companion of modern travel. With informed medical support the tourist and business man should not only be able to travel hopefully but in sound mental health.

References

Calder R and Wilder H (1989). Counselling the international traveller, *J Flor Med Assoc*, **76** 379–385

Davis K (1969). *Group Performance*, pp25–28, Addison Wesley Publishing, Massachussets

Jauhar P and Weller M (1982). Psychiatric morbidity and time zone changes, *Br J Psych*, **140** 321–325.

Lucas G E (1987). Psychological aspects of travel, *Travel Med Intl*, 99–104

McIntosh I (1990). Safe travel in the old, *Care of the Elderly*, **2.1**, 21–24.

McIntosh I (1980) Phobias, incidents, management and treatment, *Pharm Med*, **1.2**, 77–82

McIntosh I (1991). Travel Induced Illness, *Scot Med*, **11**, 14–15.

Pollitt J (1986) The mind in travel, *Trav Med Intl*, 72–74

Waterhouse J (1992). Physiological Aspects of Travel, *Update* **192**, 6

CHAPTER 4

TRAVEL PHOBIAS

Summary

Travel phobias affect many people who avoid exposure to acute anxiety by avoidance of travel. Dominant fears of travel by air or sea are commonplace and some travellers will avoid train travel for fear of traversing tunnels or bridges. Fear of heights, water, the dark, enclosed spaces and flying can all deter intending travellers from making a foreign journey. The predominance of air travel makes it likely that longer international journeys will be by aircraft. This possibility fills the phobic with apprehension and dread. Pressure from spouse, family and friends, intent on a holiday in the sun or a visit to distant relatives, often makes these individuals agree to a commercial flight against their innermost reservations. As departure day draws near, however, the phobia surfaces and anxiety intensifies. Some become so fearful that they cancel bookings. Others, under intense pressure to make the trip from fellow voyagers, present tardily to the family doctor desperate for help to calm or cure the affliction. Given enough time, much can now be done for these unfortunate people. Tranquillisers should be avoided and recourse made to behaviour therapy which can bring cure for many or make the journey an acceptable possibility for the others.

Travel fears and flying phobias in particular are common, but with good management the disabling fear, disturbed conditioned responses and frantic avoidance behaviour can be replaced by rational activity. Early and appropriate treatment will permit fearful and phobic travellers to journey free from acute anxiety.

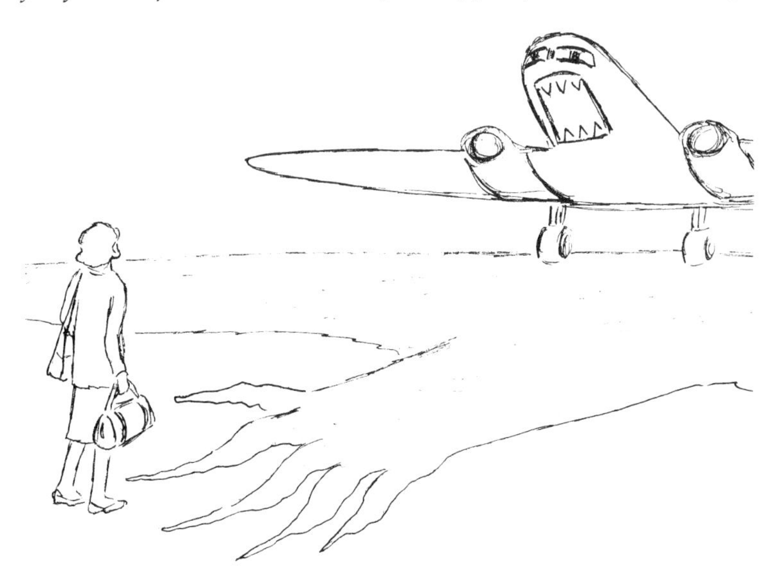

Figure 4.1: Flying Phobias
Recurrent news of mishaps and accidents to aircraft make many travellers apprehensive and fearful of flying, a condition which most overcome by rationalisation, thought-blocking or a pre-flight visit to the bar in the departure lounge. Many people, however, have a phobia for flying. This can make air travel for the business executive an absolute misery and converts holiday and social air travel for others into a severe trial and tribulation. Many feed the phobia by avoiding air travel, although the condition responds well to therapy.

Presentation

Avoidance often results in inconvenience to the individual concerned and the accompanying traveller, and can lead to family and marital conflict. Typically, the phobic presents to the family doctor a few days before a long-planned flight to a popular holiday resort. Months previously the family have convinced mum or dad that they can overcome a reluctance to fly and the vacation is arranged. As the time for departure draws ever closer, apprehension increases with anticipation and shortly before the dread day it becomes apparent to the patient that he or she cannot face the perceived ordeals of an air passage. An acute anxiety state results which reaches crisis proportions as the family becomes keyed up for departure.

Table 4.1 Anxiety and phobia

Overlapping syndromes:		
Generalised anxiety		
Anxiety and panic attacks		
Panic	—phobic situational	
	—spontaneous situational	
	—spontaneous non-situational	
Simple or social phobia	—with	panic attacks
	—without	
Agoraphobia without panic		
Agoraphobia with panic		

Alternatively, the person travelling regularly on business finds it ever more difficult to board the aircraft and goes to considerable lengths, using car, coach and train, to avoid exposure to flying. A busy schedule does not always allow for such time-consuming diversion and the phobia begins to interfere with work ability and can threaten continuation of employment.

It may be an annoying inconvenience or a severe disability and its prevalence is not well documented. As a specific phobia it can be categorised as a simple one which may be associated with panic reaction, part of a wider-ranging agoraphobia, or a major phobic disorder and, occasionally, it can be a symptom of a depressive state. Travel can involve fear of enclosed spaces , being locked in an unable to get out (in aeroplanes and ships), fear of heights, fear of water and may even include social phobias, eg. fear of eating in public and agoraphobia

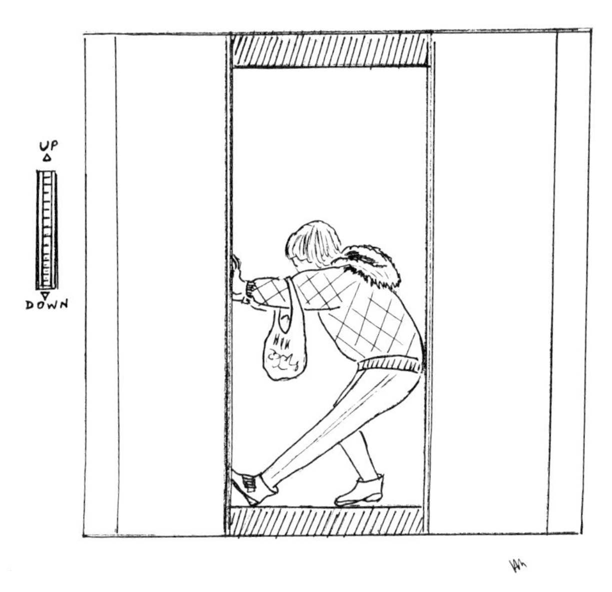

Fear of enclosed spaces

A majority of female phobics

Research

Despite surveys by Agras (1969) in the United States, Marks (1969) and Burns (1977) in Britain, there is still a marked lack of empirically based information on the prevalence of specific phobias in adults in the general population. The majority of phobics appear to be women although it is recognised that women are more likely to report their fears than men. Wilson (1967) and Burns record that travel phobias represented 2.81 percent of phobias reported by women in one survey. In a 10 percent random sample of 7074 patients in my own general medical practice (McIntosh 1980) based on a structured questionnaire listing 13 common fear-provoking objects or situations, 16 percent admitted to having a phobia and 13 percent of this sub-group reported fear of flying with a female to male preponderance of 2:1. The increase in air travel over the last decade is likely to be associated with an increase in such phobias as more people are exposed to requirements and opportunities for flying.

Disproportionate reaction

Fear is, of course, a normal and essential condition of everyday living. It is a response to a real or imagined threat with a behavioural element which is often pronounced. Minor fears are within the cultural norm and there is a continuum between mild and intense fears with the last usually described as phobia. This is considered a morbid response, disproportionate to the causative stimulus. Sufferers often structure their lives to avoid fear-provoking situations.

The phobic reaction is totally out of proportion to the situational trigger, is involuntary and cannot be explained or reasoned away by the individual involved. It leads to incapacitating avoidance behaviour and it is likely that there are many more people with flying phobias than the statistics suggest, as most simply avoid any likelihood of exposure to air travel. Those with such a condition have an irrational, uncontrollable fear resulting in avoidance behaviour which may disturb life-style and ruin opportunities for advancement.

To understand the phobic's reactions one has to consider the cognitive, physiological and behavioural components involved. The psychic element appears as overt anxiety and an exaggerated arousal response when exposed to the feared situation or even consideration of exposure, eg. as the day of the dreaded flight draws closer. The physiological response results in a sweating, tremulous, palpitating and breathless patient with assorted pains from muscle tension. The primeval fight or flight reflexes poorly prepared such people for today's flight demands.

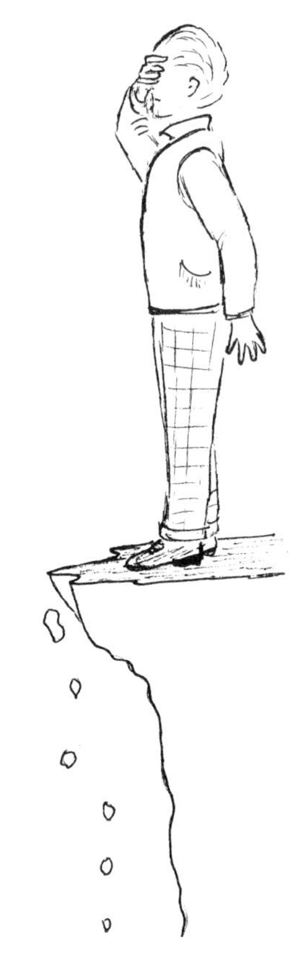

Fear of heights

Table 4.2 Fears and phobias

Phobia:
Degree of anxiety and fear out of all proportion to evoking situation
Cannot be explained or reasoned away
Beyond voluntary control
Leads to avoidance

Avoiding behaviour by the travelling executive or salesman, or the housewife's refusal to contemplate air travel thus depriving her family of a holiday in the sun, introduces a social element which often, finally, forces the patient to seek professional help.

Table 4.3 Components occurring in phobic states

Cognitive element	—person is subjectively afraid
Behavioural response	—avoidance of feared situation
Physiological manifestation which often lead to:	—tachycardia; hyperventilation
A social component	—disruption of normal living

Freudian approach

This model of a phobia helps towards a useful understanding of the problem and provides a practical approach to appropriate therapy. The vicious phobic cycle is open to curative intervention at three levels through different components. Relaxation can be taught to control physical symptoms, cognitive therapy helps to control and change fear-provoking thoughts and exposure treatment can help to overcome the restrictions in lifestyle.

In most cases, it is not known how a phobia has developed. Sometimes there is a clear cut trigger such as an unhappy incident occurring on a flight or to an aircraft before or after travel. Some are simply conditioned fear reactions. It is likely that we are more genetically predisposed to make fearful links with some situations and objects than with others; as humans we are phylogenetically prepared to learn certain stimulus responses rather than alternatives. A Freudian approach to the condition would accept that, when someone shows fear of something he knows to be harmless, then the phobic object or situation is associated with or symbolises something else that is genuinely dangerous. Freud believed that the inner conflict in such a case is then repressed and repressive aspects of it are displaced on to alternative external objects symbolising the repressed complex.

These theoretical considerations are often irrelevant to the physician who is suddenly presented with a distraught family clamouring for mother to be cured in time for the flight to Majorca a mere two days away. There is also intense pressure for immediate therapy from the businessman, whose phobia has reached such a dimension that his employment is about to be terminated due to his use of alternative and slower means of transport rather than speedy air travel; or the academic who is unexpectedly required to leave the safety of the campus to lecture in Cairo or Melbourne and cannot face the flight.

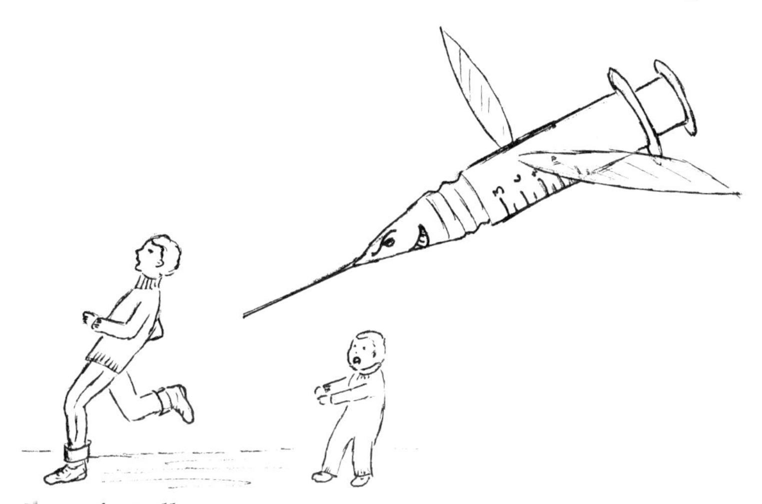

Fear of needles

Therapeutic approach

Given time, therapy can usually bring alleviation of symptoms and cure and, even at the eleventh hour, patients can be helped towards and along the frightening path from airport to aircraft and on with the flight. A phobia specific to flying can be dealt with most easily but air travel involves more than boarding the aeroplane. Crowded departure lounges will disturb the agoraphobic, the closed inescapable environment of the jet-liner frightens those with a fear of closed spaces, climbing the steps to the doorway of a jumbo jet towering above will upset those with a fear of heights, and the necessity to eat in public will cause anxiety to those with a social phobia. The need for pre-travel vaccination uncovers fear of injections. All these possibliities must be kept in mind when preparing to treat the patient who wants to make the feared flight and the even more dreaded return.

Approached at the last moment, a harassed family physician, battling through a busy surgery, will probably reach for the prescription pad and prescribe a tranquilliser. This hurried response might get the patient on to the aeroplane where, with the added boost of recourse to in-flight duty-free alcohol, the flight might just be made tolerable. The prescribed drug does nothing to cure the underlying condition, however, and merely treats the symptoms with the risk of initiating dependence upon anxiolytic drug therapy. Other therapies are available which can usually cure the patient.

Table 4.4: Phobias - management possibilities

1	Medication	benzodiazapine betablocker	} best avoided
2	Behaviour therapy	desensitisation	
3	Hypnotherapy	desensitisation flooding	

Medication

When drugs are used they ought to be prescribed for the very short term. Benzodiazepines (Tyrer 1989) are given for general anxiety, with higher dosage in anticipation of the phobic event, and the patient advised to refrain from taking alcohol or a hypnotic on the flight. Beta-blockers are used to control peripheral sympathetic responses such as palpitations. In entrenched agoraphobia with travel phobic manifestations, there is some evidence that clomipramine has an anti-phobic effect but it has to be given in high dosages. Any anti-depressant may well lift a specific phobia which has been a symptom of an underlying depression.

Behaviour therapy

Given time before the need to travel, behaviour modification is widely used in clinics to treat phobics (Marks 1975). The principle is to expose the patient to the situation which causes distress until he or she is used to it and attempts are then made to extinguish the fear by relating it to a pattern of response which provokes no anxiety. The problem behaviour needs detailed study in order to arrive at a hypothesis about its genesis and identify appropriate intervention.

Desensitisation (France and Robson 1986) consists of two features; muscle relaxation and reduction of anxiety, and the construction of a graded hierarchy of aversive stimuli from information provided by the patient. Such a hierarchy for a flying phobia would consist of arrival at the airport, proceeding to the departure lounge, walking on to the plane, experiencing take-off and landing. The hierarchy can be presented to the patient, either in imagery or in reality, and film and tape-recordings can be used effectively in desensitisation. Treatment can be assisted by vicarious or **participant modelling**. Here the therapist approaches the feared object or situation and demonstrates his confident response to it before asking the patient to do likewise. This procedure has three functions; the model encourages new patterns of behaviour to be adopted, unnecessary responses are inhibited or disinhibited and the expression of already established responses can be facilitated.

Desensitisation works well with social and specific phobias. British Airways and several universities and hospitals have run courses for phobic travellers with success. These often culminate in a short flight round the local town to demonstrate to the sufferer that the phobia has been extinguished. The disadvantage is that the process is time-consuming and often requires many sessions. Desensitisation can be carried out, however, with minimal therapist contact using tape-recordings and book instruction on relaxation and desensitisation procedures.

Another technique called flooding or **implosion** can be used to treat the phobic. If desensitisation is like wading slowly into a swimming pool at the shallow end, flooding is equivalent to jumping in at the deep end. Flooding is a prolonged exposure to the phobic situation with exposure usually initiated by flooding in fantasy with people imaging themselves in the frightening situation for one or two hours. The basic principle is to encourage the patient to face his fears rather than to avoid them. Flooding can be used very effectively with hypnosis which is possibly the most reliable method for removing the phobia when time before travel is at a premium.

Case history 4.1:

A patient telephoned in despair two days before her flight to South Africa. Having experienced recent business failure and a marriage disaster she had decided on a fresh start in a new land and was about to emigrate. With her business gone, house sold and furniture en route, her eyes were set on a new life and waiting job. All was set for the flight to Johannesburg. However, as the day for departure drew closer an inherent fear of flying which she had conquered for short flights to London resurfaced. Her thoughts had become dominated by anxiety about boarding the aeroplane. She was now proposing to cancel the air tickets and was seeking an alternative means of passage.

Despairing friends had suggest hypnosis might help her symptoms. With only two days before departure there was scant time for therapy but she pleaded for treatment and with marked reservations I arranged an appointment for that evening. She arrived in an acutely anxious state, hands never still, fingers playing with rings and pouring out a torrent of words. She said she was petrified at the prospect of entering the narrow confines of the aircraft.

In discussion it became obvious that her unspoken doubts were about her proposed changed life situation far from her homeland. All her misgivings were being channelled to acute apprehension focussed into the imminent air travel.

She had refused medication from her GP on the grounds that many years before she had become dependent upon hypnotics and did not now want to take drugs. There was little time for behavioural deconditioning and the only recourse was hypnotherapy. She proved to be a good subject and easily entered a trance-state wherupon ego-strengthening and relaxation techniques were offered to her and she was left with post-hypnotic suggestions that flight and emigration would be accomplished successfully. This procedure was repeated on the evening before the flight and she was encouraged to visually hallucinate her progression through the airport, emigration control and on to the plane while maintaining a relaxed state. She became very agitated at the envisaged point of entry to the aircraft but with further relaxation managed to continue the hallucinatory progress without further abreaction.

Next day she made a successful flight. A year later she sent a grateful letter with news of a highly profitable business venture in South Africa and a successful transition to her adopted country.

Hypnosis therapy

The use of hypnosis for phobias (McIntosh 1981) borrows both from behaviour modification and desensitisation but therapy is facilitated by induction of a tranced state.

Teaching the patient auto-hypnosis, whereby at a coded signal he or she can recreate the relaxed state acquired at earlier sessions, decreases the risk of dependence and diminishes the time required for therapy. Graded desensitisation and flooding are both practicable within the trance-states and visual imagery and vicarious modelling can also be used. A modified flooding technique is used and it is very effective for specific phobias such as flying (McIntosh 1991).

Case history 4.2

One of my patients, who had patiently built up his business, had a unique opportunity presented to his firm for advancement and profit in the Far East, but he had long had a phobia for air travel. Unable to resist the opportunity for expansion, he made his plans, bought his tickets, and the day before departure, succumbed to panic and terror at the thought of many hours incarcerated in an aircraft. In the surgery, he was in a state of agitation but refused to consider a drug prescription as he wished to be mentally fit for tough business negotiations upon arrival in Hong Kong.

He accepted the offer of hypnotherapy with alacrity and, proving to be a good subject, was quickly in a trance and relaxed. Soon he was able to create a visual image of himself boarding and sitting in the aeroplane and, with continued suggestion of calmness, muscle and mind relaxation and freedom from tension, he was able to fantasise himself through a prolonged exposure to the feared situation. Given post-hypnotic suggestions that he would remain calm throughout the flight, and that the standard pre-take-off and recorded music would relax him, he went off to make a successful return flight and business deal. Even when the jet-liner was buffeted badly by turbulence and suddenly dropped

500 feet, with dramatic appearance of personal passenger oxygen masks from their overhead stowage, he was able to keep calm. Now after a decade and many air trips he remains undisturbed by his once disabling phobia.

Gentle words

'Gentle words, quiet words are after all the most powerful words. They are more convincing, more compelling, more prevailing and successful'. So wrote a patient on return from her first successful air trip after years of phobic avoidance. However, the removal of psychosomatic symptoms before the patient is ready, and has built up more socially satisfactory defences, can precipitate more serious difficulties. Therapists have to keep this in mind. It seems likely, however, that desensitisation can be carried out with little therapist contact using tape-recordings to carry out relaxation and desensitisation procedures. These are a useful adjuvant in desensitisation and hypnotherapy. Book and computer instruction courses offering graded and detailed programmes of relaxation and exposure are available, and have proved of value to many phobics.

Conclusion

Although phobias of air travel and flying are common and likely to become more prevalent, the phobic air traveller need not despair as there are thriving phobic societies, several books and many therapists trained to offer support and guidance. With good management and encouragement from the doctor at a conventional consultation or at a travel health clinic, the disabling fear, disturbed conditioned responses and frantic avoidance behaviour can be replaced by rational activity and more normal, socially acceptable reactions and conditioned responses.

References

Agras S, Sylvester D and Oliveau D (1969). The epidemiology of common fears and phobias. *Comprehensive Psych*, **10:2**, 151.
Burns L, Thorpe G (1977). Fears and Phobias, *J Intnl Med R*es, **5** Suppl 1, 132–139.
France R, Robson M (1986). *Behaviour therapy in primary care*, p66, Croom Helm
Marks I (1975). *Progress in behaviour therapy*, Academic Press, New York.
McIntosh, I (1980). Incidence, management and treatment of phobias in a group medical practice, *Pharm Med*, **1:2**, 77–82.
McIntosh I (1981). Hypnotherapy: The case for the GP, *Psych Pract*, November 1981.
McIntosh I (1991). Treating travel phobias with hypmotherapy, *J Brit Socy Med & Dent Hypnosis*, **7.5**, 18-21.
Tyrer P (1989). Treating Panic, *Br Med J*, **298**, 201.
Wilson G (1967). Social desirability and sex differences in expressed fear, *Behav Res Ther*, **5**, 136.

Recommended reading

Marks I (1978). *Living With Fear*, McGraw Hill, Maidenhead.
Mitchell R (1982). *Phobias*, Penguin Books, London.
Steptoe A, (1988). Managing flying phobia, *Br Med J*, **296**, 1756-1757.

CHAPTER 5

TRAVEL SICKNESS

Summary

Many people dare not travel for fear of succumbing to the miseries of motion illness. They cannot travel upon or around the planet without suffering the consequences of an unstable environment. High-flying modern jets soaring through clear skies, stabilised passenger ships and broad, gently curving motorways have diminished the incidence of travel sickness. Many travellers, however, still suffer, in greater or lesser degree, from this disabling malady. Anticipatory drug therapy can provide a measure of protection with manageable side-effects but the world still waits for the ideal anti-motion remedy.

Motion sickness is a debilitating but relatively short-lived illness which indiscriminately affects air, land and sea travellers. This malady has attracted much investigation recently, with the advent of cosmic travel and its attendant space-sickness. It appears to have affected man through recorded time. It was certainly well known to ancient Greek seafarers who referred to it as nauxia - sea-sickness — the precursor of the English word, nausea. Greek mythology records that the fair maiden, Helle, flying home from her adventures on a golden ram, was affected by vertigo and inadvertently fell into the sea giving to it the name of the Hellespont. Julius Caesar apparently suffered grievously from the disease on his crossing of the Channel and the illustrious Admiral Lord Nelson had to fight sea-sickness before his battles against sea-borne invaders.

Significant problems

Despite much study, there are still no reliable predictive tests of individual susceptibility to motion sickness and no perfect counter-measures – or remedies to counter its onset.

The textbooks refer to travel sickness as a physiological vertigo and the autonomic symptoms are all too familiar to many. The onset follows a variable sequence of drowsiness, yawning, cold sweats, increased salivation and general malaise. Associated with epigastric discomfort, nausea and pallor, digestion is impaired and the sight or smell of food aggravates the condition which proceeds like an avalanche to vomiting and varying degrees of apathy, depression and incapacity.

Table 5.1: Autonomic symptoms of Travel Sickness

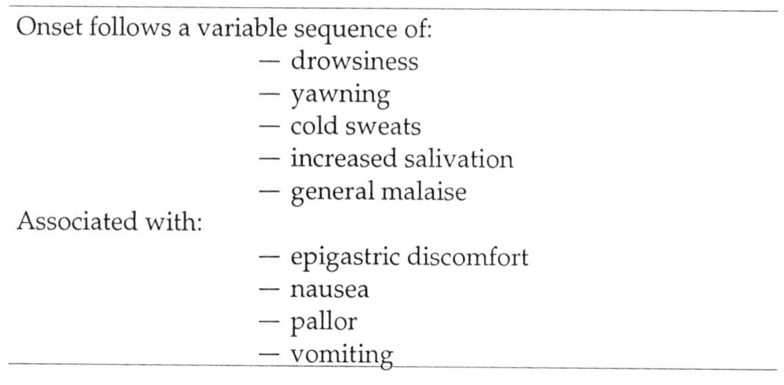

Onset follows a variable sequence of:	
	— drowsiness
	— yawning
	— cold sweats
	— increased salivation
	— general malaise
Associated with:	
	— epigastric discomfort
	— nausea
	— pallor
	— vomiting

Circulatory, respiratory and psychological disturbance are often apparent. Hyperventilation is common, leading to hypocapnia and changes in blood volume, with pooling in the lower parts of the body accompanied by postural hypotension and syncope.

Variability of symptoms

Symptoms can be present in variable degree, may wax and wane but develop over time and steadily worsen with exposure to the environmental instability. New cases continue to appear after many hours, as unaccustomed motion continues. Characteristically, vomiting eases the symptoms temporarily but persistent vomiting over several days of travel can often result in dehydration and electrolyte imbalance. Females are more susceptible to motion sickness than males, with a reported adult male to female incidence of 2:5 (Nicholson 1992).

With professional aviators and seamen, a significant factor is the effect on performance as 60 to 80 percent of sailors in naval off-shore patrol boats have been shown to suffer sea-sickness in rough weather. Many become unfit to continue conventional duties. Pilots, on holding patterns in turbulent air conditions, become air-sick with possible hazardous effects on performance. Most airline company regulations preclude use of anti-motion medication.

Cause

The exact cause of motion-sickness is still not understood, but the illness arises from stimulation of the labyrinthine sense organs over a lengthy period, in an intense manner to which the body is not accustomed. The condition only occurs in those with intact labyrinths. It is, perhaps, related to conflicting information in brain input from the visual and labyrinthine sensors, which is then read in relation to a pattern of expected associations stored in the brain. The brain's failure to match perceived and received information results in conflict, dissonance and physiological disturbance.

Many believe that the emetic chemoreceptor trigger zone in the area postrema of the medulla oblongata is incriminated in producing motion-illness. It has been postulated that, due to motion a vomiting substance is secreted into the cerebrospinal fluid in the emetic process and that therapeutic measures should be directed at prevention of its secretion. Borison (1985), however, concludes from overall evidence that the area postrema is not essential for motion-induced vomiting and it is irrational to seek pharmacological blocking-agents that act at the chemoreceptor trigger zone. He believes that an as yet unidentified neural element indispensable for motion-induced vomiting is located close to the area postrema. Identification of this feature and its neurochemical links could be the breakthrough required for an effective therapy for motion sickness.

Habituation

A striking feature of motion sickness is individual ability to become accustomed to motion. Most people habituate to the adverse stimulus over time but the conditioning is lost when exposure is discontinued and re-exposure is delayed. Habituation is also related to the pattern of motion with travellers in large ships becoming ill on transferring to small ones whilst sailors can become air-sick when transferring to aircraft exposed to sustained turbulence. The change in ability to withstand the disturbing stimuli presumably includes a learning component with the individual adapting postural control and locomotor function to the moving environment.

Simulator machines are often used to test for propensity to motion sickness although there have been occasions when cosmonauts most resistant to rotational stimulation have succumbed markedly to space-sickness in flight.

Machines have shown that the frequency of up and down movement most likely to induce illness is one cycle in 16 seconds. Frequencies higher than one cycle per second produce little motion sickness. The study of autonomic response in motion sickness stimulation has shown increases in pulse rate, ventilation and vasoconstriction and provided data to support the supposition that motion illness can be categorised as a stress reaction (Cowing and Suter 1986).

Prevention

Only deaf-mutes with non-functioning labyrinths are known to be immune to the malady. The use of stabilisers on large ships diminishes the incidence of the disease. Assuming the horizontal position is a useful preventive measure as it removes vertical acceleration, a dominant component of the disturbance. Keeping the head fixed relative to the body, maintaining the eyes on the horizon and avoiding fixating on proximal moving stimuli is also useful in prevention. Involvement in physical work on board ship, but avoiding reading, is also helpful and many of those who are car-sick as passengers will be aware that they can avoid succumbing to the illness by driving themselves. Stuffy atmospheres and smells of cooking and fuel oil are stimuli likely to induce vomiting and should also be avoided.

Those who have suffered the trauma of travel-sickness will testify to the need for an effective preventive or remedy. The toughest and fittest can succumb.

Case history 5.1

I recall an occasion when as medical officer I was accompanying a high climbing expedition of brawny mountaineers en route to

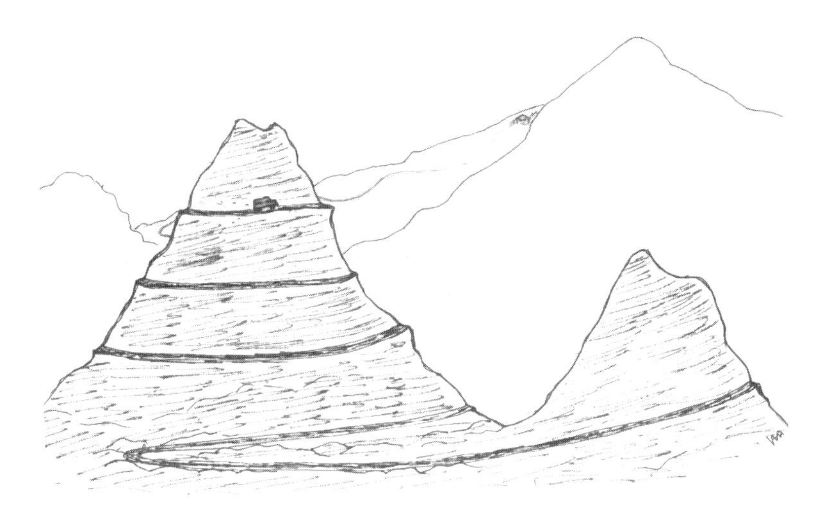

Travel-sickness

the Himalayas. Engine problems had grounded the scheduled jet service to Nepal and we transferred to an ancient piston-driven aeroplane for the flight over the hump to Kathmandu. Turbulent air space over the foothills had the aircraft bouncing and pitching as it clawed its way to higher altitude and tough 'tigers of the tops' were soon devastated by air sickness. Some were prostrated; once suntanned faces took on an unaccustomed pallor and several became green of visage as nausea and vomiting took their toll.

Drug therapy

Drug therapy can be prophylactic but there is a strong placebo effect with anti-motion therapy. Controlled studies have shown that up to 55 percent of a group can benefit from appropriate drug provision but 45 percent will benefit from placebo. Anti-motion drugs are not very effective in diminishing symptoms once the condition is established. They can provide protection during the first three to five days of exposure to vestibular stimulation, and habituation usually progressively increases to provide protection after this initial period.

1-Hyoscine (Scopolamine) has been considered to be the best drug for combating motion sickness (Dahl 1984) especially for brief exposure, but has been of limited value orally and as an injection because of side-effects. The anti-nauseant effect of scopolamine does not depend upon its peripheral parasympathetic blocking capacity but is caused by a central effect.

Hyoscine has a predominant place in therapy because of its efficacy but it does suffer from side-effects. It causes a dry mouth and dilation of the pupils with resultant loss of visual acuity and it has often a 'drugging' effect which causes a relaxed state of mind and disinclination to incentive and activity. The latter is a disadvantage where immediate action and response is required. The drug only works for a short period of six to eight hours.

There is no advantage in combining an anti-histamine and hyoscine. Swallowed tablets need to be ingested an hour before exposure but some, like 'kwells ,' are absorbed quite rapidly when taken sub-lingually. A hyoscine patch is marketed which is stuck behind the ear and gives three days' protection. This is usually sufficient to allow habituation to free the victim from the disease.

Case history 5.2

I tested the efficiency of the transdermal patch on a group of tourists en route from the Indian plains to Darjeeling. In former days, a narrow gauge railway carried the colonials sedately up to this lofty hill station and into Sikkim. Landslides now block the railway and a narrow congested road spirals upwards in stomach-churning twists and turns. Many tourists arrive in Darjeeling nauseated and prostrated from vehicle sickness. My fellow travellers wearing the patch were effectively protected from the ravages of motion sickness.

Hyoscine tablet dosage is two 0.3mg of the hypobromide taken an hour before travel and followed up at intervals of eight hours to a limit of 2mg per 24 hours. This can give up to 90 percent protection from vomiting but combats the nausea to a lesser extent.

The antihistamines are popular although not as effective as hyoscine. Using the transdermal route of administration allows delivery of the drug in an effective concentration in a dosage low enough to avoid severe adverse reactions. The efficacy of transdermally adminstered scopolamine has been compared with the efficacy of dimenhydrinate and placebo in a double-blind controlled study. The patch afforded 61–67 percent protection against motion sickness at sea against 48–88 percent protection from dimenhydrinate. Dry mouth is the main side-effect reported for the patch, occurring in around two-thirds of users. Temporary blurring of vision may also occur with the drug which is otherwise well tolerated in transdermal presentation. The patch also has the advantage that it can be removed if the need for protection becomes no longer paramount. They do give longer protection for up to 72 hours but cause sedation as a side-effect. This can be welcomed by the traveller confronted by a tedious journey but is potentially hazardous for those involved in decision-making and transport control.

Promethazine (Phenergan) and cyclizine (marzine) are given in a dosage of 25 to 50mg in 24 hours and with a protection range of 40 to 70 percent in those treated. The use of anti-motion drugs for civil and military flyers has been resisted on the grounds that any medication or condition requiring medication is likely to diminish operational proficiency to a dangerous level. Preparatory work for space-flight travel has suggested, however, that selected dosage and combinations of promethazine, scopolamine and d-amphetamine could be used in cosmonauts without loss of operational proficiency (Wood and Manno 1985).

Management

I, personally, have found the patch ideal for prolonged car-passenger travel, and have tested its efficacy rigorously on the interminable, high-climbing circuitous, constantly-looping roads of the high Andes. Any soporific side-effects prompt towards sleep which helps to while away tedious miles of mountain travel.

Case history 5.3

Scopalamine patch prophylaxis was used by expeditioners climbing high into the Himalayas. A narrow hazardous road cork-screws into the remote kingdom of Bhutan. It climbs for thousands of feet inching upwards in a continuous series of tight convolutions, clawing forward above plunging chasms, vertiginous drops and fearsome cliffs. A day of travel is required to negotiate the passage into this mountain fortress – a day in which motion sickness often afflicts the car-bound. The unprotected succumb to severe gastric disturbance during the lengthy journey. Those in the party wearing the patch made the trip sleepily but free from symptoms of travel sickness.

Once the individual has succumbed to the illness, he or she should be encouraged to lie down, if possible, with eyes closed. The prostrated should be kept warm and given sips of water to avoid dehydration. The very ill over a longer period may require enteral or parenteral fluids. Despite the misery of the condition while it lasts most people, on a longer journey, can expect substantial improvement over a day or two. A remarkable feature is the self limitation of effects and the rapidity of recovery once motion ceases.

Instructions for Patients

Sea-sickness

1. Anticipate the event and apply a transdermal hyoscine skin patch three to four hours before starting the voyage
2. Keep in the fresh air as much as possible
3. Fix the eyes on the horizon
4. Keep the head fixed in relation to the body
5. Lie down if symptoms seem imminent, with the head towards the centre of rotation and close eyes.

Car-sickness

1. A short-acting preventive (eg. Kwells) may suffice but must be taken one hour before travel.
2. Use a head-rest to fix the head position.
3. Open fresh-air vents and windows to avoid a hot, stuffy atmosphere.
4. Fix eyes on the distant view or keep them closed.

Air-sickness

1. Long flights merit the use of the transdermal hyoschine patch, applied behind the ear before arrival at the airport.
2. Avoid ingesting alcohol.
3. Eat little.
4. Keep the head fixed against the headrest.

References

Borison L (1985). *Aviation, Space and Environmental Medicine* **56,** 66–68.
Cowing S, Suter S *et al* (1986). *Psychophysiology,* **23** 542–551.
Dahl E *et al* (1984). *Clinical Pharmacology and Therapeutics,* **36,** 116–119
Nicholson P J (1992). *Physiological factors and the female pilot,* **10.2,** 68-71
Wood D, Manno L *et al* (1985). *Aviation, Space and Environmental Medicine,* **56,** 310–315.

CHAPTER 6

THE CHILD TRAVELLER

Summary

Many potential health hazards can befall the young traveller. Awareness of risk, pre-travel medical consultation, vaccination, prophylaxis and counselling should ensure that a child can travel the world healthily and successfully.

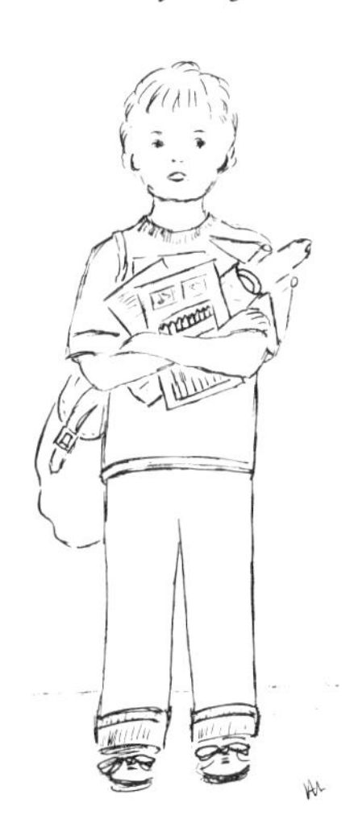

Figure 6.1: Child Traveller

World travel is now undertaken by the young and old, children and infants often circumnavigating the globe. Older children travel as immigrants, tourists and adventurers to remote places and do so with remarkable success and in safety. Adaptable and devoid of racial and colour bias, children often bridge cultural and linguistic barriers in a manner denied accompanying adults. International travel is not, however, devoid of health risks for the young and very young.

Naivety, ignorance and inquisitive exploratory behaviour can add to the usual risks of travel-induced illness which can befall older voyagers. Children and early teenagers may succumb rapidly to infections which are only a nuisance to older individuals. Sensible precautions, instigated at pre-travel medical consultation, can help towards safe world transit and foreign sojourns for small travellers.

Planning

Assessment has to consider age, destination, living abode, planned route, duration of stay, types of transport and holiday involved. Travelling with children is undoubtedly stressful to accompanying adults and adds to the conventional psychological hazards of any global relocation (Lucas 1987). Careful parental planning before the vacation can minimise health hazards and travel disturbance when travelling abroad with children. The unfamiliarity of the milieu met in global travel tends to knit families closer together. Tightened family bonds, in bigger groups, alleviate much of the potential psychological upset which can affect the only child exposed to traumatic relocation.

Management

Baby feeding

Babies travel relatively well with the breast-fed more easily managed en route and abroad than those fed by bottle on a formula (Travelling Health 1991). Maternal inhibitions about feeding in public may have to be overcome but acceptance may be easier in countries abroad where public breast-feeding is the cultural norm.

Breast-feeding can ensure an uncontaminated food and water supply for small babies and, even in very hot countries, there is no need to supplement with water, providing the mother maintains a high fluid input. Even if the mother has contracted an infection, with most diseases breast-feeding remains safe for the baby. Feeding schedules may have to be altered and feeding routines can be disturbed during travel with the bottle-fed. A hungry, bawling infant does not make the ideal travelling companion. Bottle and formulary-fed babies are at higher risk of receiving contaminated feeds during foreign travel. Pre-packed milk is a wise provision for the journey and meticulous attention to sterility is vital while overseas. Milk and water supplies may well be infected outside northern Europe, North America, Australia and New Zealand.

Pressure changes

Changes in air pressure can cause eustachian problems in babies during air travel but these are usually alleviated if the child cries during ascent and descent. The problem can be more serious if a virus infection has already produced a stuffy nose and older babies may benefit from a small dosage of an antihistamine before the journey. The sedative side-effect may also be calming during the flight.

Immunization

Babies ought to receive conventional vaccinations within normal schedules for diphtheria, pertussis, poliomyelitis and tetanus before departure. These vaccinations can be undertaken from the age of two months. BCG can be given at birth or any age in infancy if the risk of tuberculosis is high in the country to be visited. Infants over six months and young children can be submitted to the full range of vaccinations and also to anti-malarials. The latter are prescribed in reduced dosages and newer preparations are not recommended until five years. Cholera, yellow fever, hepatitis A and typhoid vaccine should only be given after six months. Protective control measures against mosquitoes, such as nets and room sprays, will be necessary from birth in the absence of anti-malarial drug protection for the very young.

Travel Travail

Young children are remarkable resilient to the hassle of relocation and will often sleep through the tiresome delays inseparable from modern travel. Bored children are, however, a travail for parents and fellow travellers, and toys to hold attention, books and diversions are prerequisites in planning children's travel. A fractious, obstreperous child on a protracted aircraft or train journey is a source of embarrassment to all around. Irritability may be compounded by disturbance in circadian rhythm with time-zone transitions and the use of a mild sedative may well be necessary. Promethazine, five to 10 mg for the one to five year-old and 10 to 25 mg for those over five, may be advantageous. The side-effect of sleepiness is beneficial in long-haul travel. Once asleep, most children will be unaffected by environmental disturbance. Most airlines provide a well-organised service for unaccompanied older children who are packaged round the world with consummate ease.

Table 6.1 Children' immunizations for far flung holidays

Disease		0–5 yrs	5–10 yrs	10+yrs
Cholera*	First dose	1.1ml	0.3ml	0.5ml
	Second dose and booster	0.3ml	0.5ml	1.0ml
Typhoid*	First dose	0.25ml	0.25ml	0.5ml
	Second dose and booster	0.25ml	0.25ml	0.5ml
Yellow fever†		0.5ml from 9 months of age		
Meningitis		Single dose of 0.5ml from 2 months of age		
Hepatitis A (immuno-globulin)	If abroad for:			
	2 months or less	125mg	125mg	250mg
	3–5 months	250mg	250mg	500mg
(Hepatitis A Vaccination only for over 16 yr olds)				
Hepatitis B	Using Engerix	0.5ml	0.5ml (1ml if over 12)	0.5ml

*Not recommended under 12 months
†Not recommended under 9 months

Credit: Dr Nick Cooper, MIMS Magazine, July 1991

Travel-sickness

Travel-sickness is the bane of many infant travellers. Vehicle-sickness can affect cot-bound infants with the accompanying risk of inhalation of vomitus which can go unobserved. Positioning the cot in line with direction of travel decreases the incidence of vestibular disturbance. Younger children prone to motion-sickness should be discouraged from reading, placed on a raised cushion in

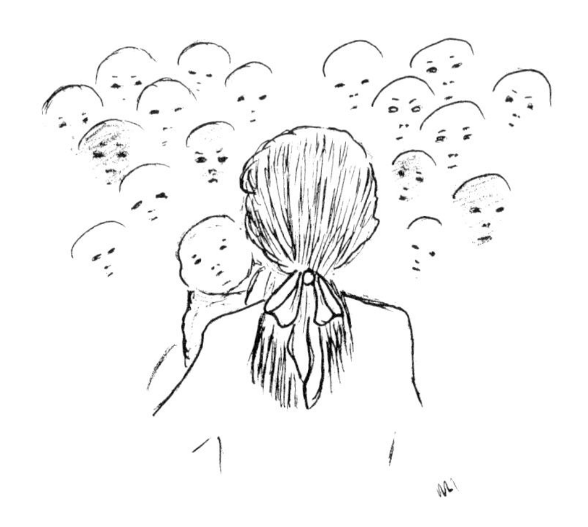

Travelling with children

the front seat of a car and encouraged to look forward during travel. Sadly, looking at the view rapidly bores the child and nausea is likely to intervene. Most children benefit from an anti-emetic given in small dosages in advance of the trip.

Prochlorperazine syrup 0.25 mg/kg for those weighing more than 10 kg, although pyramidal side-effects can restrict its use.

Cinnarizine (Stugeron) 7.5 mg two hourly before travel then eight hourly during the journey is appropriate for those over five years. Sleepiness is a side-effect which can be a travel aid but associated irritability and a dry mouth often upset children and bring constant complaints.

Repeated requests for drinks are difficult to contain during travel as too much fluid may bring more vomiting. Only deaf mutes, with non-functioning labyrinths are known to be immune to travel sickness (McIntosh 1990).

Table 6.2: Instructions for parents of travel sick children

Have the child in the front seat of a vehicle with good ventilation
Avoid feeding a heavy meal before commencement of the journey
Prevent the child from reading or drawing in the car
Stop the vehicle at regular intervals along the way
Encourage the child to lie flat if sqeamish on sea crossings
Ensure childrens' cots are placed parallel to direction of travel
Consider anti-emetic medication prior to the journey

On sea voyages, squeamish children should be encouraged to lie flat as this removes the effects of vertical acceleration, a dominant component of vestibular disturbance associated with travel sickness. As parents are well aware, it is a major task to keep small children immobilised for any length of time except when they are asleep. Family groups determined to travel may have to accept a vomiting child as the price to be paid to reach their foreign objective.

Travellers' Diarrhoea

Having survived the vagaries of the journey, children adapt quickly to a new environment. However, curious young children who finger and mouth objects on the ground and imbibe water and food unconcerned with potential health hazards, are at greater risk than adults of contracting travellers' diarrhoea. According to one study (Travelling Healthy 1991), in the first 14 days in the tropics travellers' diarrhoea occurred in 30 percent of children under the age of two years, 8.5 percent of children between three and six years, 21.7 percent of those aged between seven and 14 years and in 33 percent of adolescents. The diarrhoea in the infants was more severe and longer lasting.

Specific and repeated instruction by the parents on the need to avoid tap water unless of known purity is essential. Parents should ensure that ice-cream, milk and bottled water is sterile before ingestion. Fruits and sweets, eaten without thought by youngsters at home, may be suspect abroad and children should be kept, forcibly, away from them.

Children's diarrhoea in tropical regions is commonly caused by a rota virus resulting in mild fever, watery diarrhoea and vomiting. *Salmonella* food poisoning and bacillary dysentery are also involved. Diarrhoea can rapidly lead to dehydration in small children, with electrolyte loss and metabolic disturbance. It requires prompt fluid and electrolyte replacement with dioralyte or rehydrat. Fortunately, most infections will settle on this regimen. Children resisting medication, will often take a coca cola or soda which has been allowed to go 'flat' as an alternative to conventional therapy.

Other infections

Hepatitis A virus is spread by the faecal-oral route and children are particularly liable to infection, with the highest incidence abroad recorded in children of school age. It often presents as diarrhoea and although mortality is low, it may cause prolonged incapacitation. Intramuscular injection of gamma globulin can be given before travel to children over six months who are visiting endemic areas. Hepatitis A vaccination (HAVRIX) is now available for those over 16 years. The risks of hepatitis B infection must also be considered.

Parents have now to recognise the risk of AIDS transmission from contaminated needles and blood transfusion equipment when calling upon primary care services in developing countries, especially in Africa. The need for sutures and injections for an injured or feverish child has to be weighed against the possibility of a health professional using infected equipment. A wise precaution is for parents to carry syringes and needles on trips to countries where the risk is high. Children are prone to chip teeth and lose cavity fillings with the resultant pain forcing recourse to emergency dental care and the risk of infection from dental needles.

Sleep

Transmeridian travel can be disturbing for juniors deprived of sleep at conventional hours and forced into altered time cycles current at the destination. The use of a 'skycot' on aircraft journeys ensures a safe environment for the baby in transit. It should be held in the arms or on the lap at take-off and landing to provide reassurance and additional support. Sleep upset, irritability and appetite change can be expected for up to a week after protracted east/west and west/east flights. Efforts to minimise circadian effects, by prompt adherence to the life cycle of the new venue on arrival, are unlikely to be appreciated by small children intent on maintaining their own routines and unprepared to take to bed at apparently inappropriate times. Jet-lag is more severe from west to east and parents are well advised to endeavour to start flights in the morning and take advantage of night stop-overs when practicable (McIntosh 1990).

Sun, sea and watersports

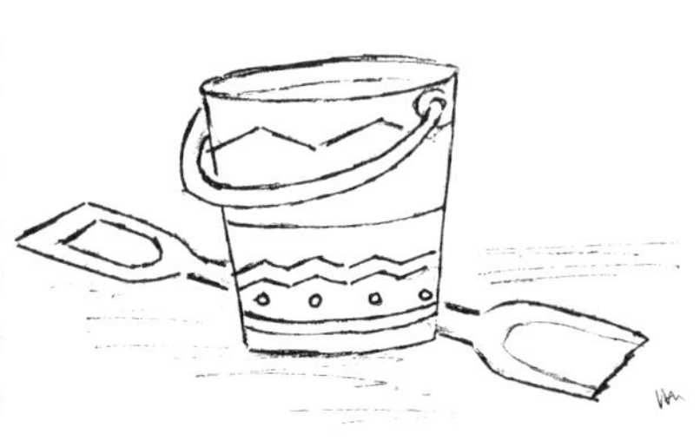

Sun-burn is a hazard, especially in fair-skinned children. At most holiday destinations short, graduated exposure, protective clothing, the use of high-factor sun screens and avoidance of exposure to the sun between 11am and 3pm are essential factors in protecting the young from severe burns. Over-exposure to ultraviolet light, with severe burning as a child, appears to be a contributory factor to malignant melanoma activity in later life. Even one acute sunburn in childhool, significantly increases subsequent risk. High altitude, the waterside, water sports and swimming activities make sunburn even more likely in children intent on play and oblivious of time.

Teenagers are unaware of risk and appropriate precautions when sporting themselves in foreign waters, and are more likely to succumb to sports injury and sports-induced infection. Few youngsters appreciate the potential dangers rife in African waters, where rivers, lakes and even hotel swimming pools may be polluted or harbour bilharzia. Even when warned of such dangers, the temptation to cool off with a swim is often irresistible.

Ear infections are common in children staying in hot countries and swimming should be avoided until well after recovery. Young teenagers break their necks and are paralysed by diving too steeply into shallow pools when on holiday. Surfing injuries are common in the novice, and surfers can also be severely injured when diving steeply into waves at the water's edge and thrusting the head on to an unsuspected sand-bank with resultant neck fracture (Grundy and Penney 1991).

In and by the sea

Freshwater swimming in many popular holiday resorts now runs the risk of a swim in sewage-polluted waters with increased risk of conjunctivitis and ear infections. Swimmers in the Mediterranean have been shown to suffer more gastro-intestinal upsets than non-swimmers. Algal bloom can contaminate fresh water lakes and children swimming in them can develop pneumonia (Dunlop 1991).

The young do not consider the possibility of bilharzia infection in much of Africa. Desperate for a swim to cool off, they plunge into infected pools, rivers and lakes. Even unmaintained swimming pools can harbour infected snails and result in swimmers' infection.

Young water-side paddlers and small toddlers risk infection from Larva migransi, the hookworm lava which inhabits beach sand and burrows into human skin, wandering at will just beneath the surface. This infection can largely be avoided by ensuring that children wear sandals on the beach. The use of beach shoes also diminishes common childhood injuries from corals (McIntosh 1991). Bare-foot walking in the tropics, always a temptation for children, brings the risk of bites from scorpions, snakes and insects. Although deaths from scorpion bites are unusual most occur in children under two years. Children have to be encouraged to cover exposed limbs at dusk to avoid malarial infection, and dissuaded from playing with strange dogs which may be rabid in Asia and Africa.

Canoeing is a favourite pastime for older children and exposure to water contaminated with rat urine can expose the canoeist to leptospirosis. Childrens' predilection for water sports exposes them to the risk of drowning or hypothermia.

High altitude

Children walking in high mountain areas can easily succumb to exposure and die quickly from hypothermia if symptoms are not spotted early. Presentation in the young is subtle and can easily be missed. The tendency to stumble, incoherent speech and excessive fatigue may be the only signs before sudden loss of consciousness. Young teenagers, exercising at high altitude, are more likely to encounter problems with acute mountain sickness than adults. When left to their own resources, they often over-exercise and climb too far, too fast and too high, and do not allow themselves to acclimatise to changes in partial pressures of oxygen.

Acetazolamide can be an effective prophylactic. Taken 24 hours before climbing over 12,000 feet and daily with ascent therafter, the drug will provide some protection. Dose is age-dependent, 500 mg sustet daily is appropriate for those over 12 years of age.

Despite the many potential hazards which can befall the young, most travel the globe in safety and many parents who have taken children to remote parts do so without incident. Children can be an asset as travel companions and in some countries, such as China with its one family/one child policy, they are almost venerated. Unaware of race and colour barriers, they quickly make friends with other children and facilitate contact with local people. With appropriate vaccination, precautionary education, awareness of risks and a watchful, parental eye, most will travel the world successfully and safely. They should develop a wealth of environmental and cultural experience of inestimable value to them in later life.

References

Dunlop G (1991). Blooming algae, *Br Med J*, **286,** 1337–9.
Editorial (1991). *Travelling Healthy*, **4**; 4,4, Travel Health Inc, New York.
Grundy D, Penney P *et al* (1991) Diving into the unknown, *Br Med J*, **302** 670–1.
Lucas G E (1987). Psychological aspects of travel. *Travel Med Intl*, 99–104.
McIntosh I (1991). Health hazards and water sports abroad, *Travel Med Intl*, 126–130.
McIntosh I (1990). Travel sickness, *Travel Med Intl*, 180.
McIntosh I (1990). The stress of modern travel, *Travel Med Intl*, 118–121.
Walker E and Williams G (1983). ABC of healthy travel, *Br Med J*, **286**, 1337–1339.

CHAPTER 7

THE WOMAN TRAVELLER

Summary

World travel has never been the prerogative of the male. Intrepid women have long ventured to the far corners of the earth and proved themselves equal to man in world exploration They have demonstrated an ability to withstand hostile terrain, climatic and environmental extremes and remain in sound health. There are, however, medical, psychological and cultural aspects of global travel which the potential female traveller should consider before embarking on long adventurous journeys, especially if the intention is to travel alone. Before departure, many women approach family doctors for advice regarding immunisations, prophylaxis and health precautions, and the informed doctor should be able to tailor advice to the individual and her itinerary.

Early women travellers

In 353 AD, the Roman noblewoman Egeria journeyed from Gaul to Palestine, recording her experiences of conflict with wild animals, wily natives and aggressive bandits intent on robbery and rape. En route, she suffered from severe enteritis, the scourge of travellers through the ages, but according to Jerome, a contemporary writer, she forgot her sex and physical weakness in the determination to travel independently to her goal. She was the first of many female pilgrims to tread the route to the Holy Land. By the 8th century, the pilgrim's way had become a tourist trail. It was followed by so many that the Church attempted to stem the tide of restless women, seeing them as an evil influence, unrestrained by the institution of marriage and marital fidelity.

In 1413, there is a record of an English Mayor's daughter setting off by sea to travel independently to Jerusalem and treating her sea-sickness en route with herbs. She often trudged alone over foreign tracks, combating the loneliness and isolation of the single traveller by recourse to prayer. By the 18th century, waves of women travellers were following their husbands to diplomatic posts across the world. Spinsters embarked on travel in the guise of missionaries, one of the few travel roles permitted to them by society. In the missionary field, they were thought to present no threat to the local populace, and they were expected to pursue their religious objectives while disregarding bodily discomfort, dangers and alien climes. Religious fervour was deemed to overcome physical exhaustion, lack of sustenance, isolation and ill-health. They tolerated ridicule, humiliation, rejection and physical and sexual harassment, sustained by their religious beliefs and the determination to venture with man into the unknown.

First female ascent of Mont Blanc

Victorian women travellers performed feats of endurance beset and constrained by the cultural mores and morality of the times. When Mary Kingsley set off for West Africa she fully expected to die there. She was advised to make early contact with the Wesleyan missionaries as that would provide her only chance of a decent burial with a hearse and black feathers.

The first female ascent of Mont Blanc was made by a woman wearing a long ankle-length skirt which she hitched up over borrowed male trousers when climbing. Despite the voluminous, thick and long skirts worn by Victorian ladies visiting the Holy Land, they recorded sexual harassment from 'pint-sized bottom pinchers' who jostled them in the souks.

The 20th century has seen women disputing male domination in world exploration and ultimately notching up an impressive array of travel firsts. They have often done so despite social condemnation, male disapproval and sexual intimidation. Women travellers have overcome the boredom, fear, loneliness, physical and psychological discomfiture inseparable from international travel to remote places. Their adventures have exploded the myth of an inherent female weakness in the face of environmental extremes.

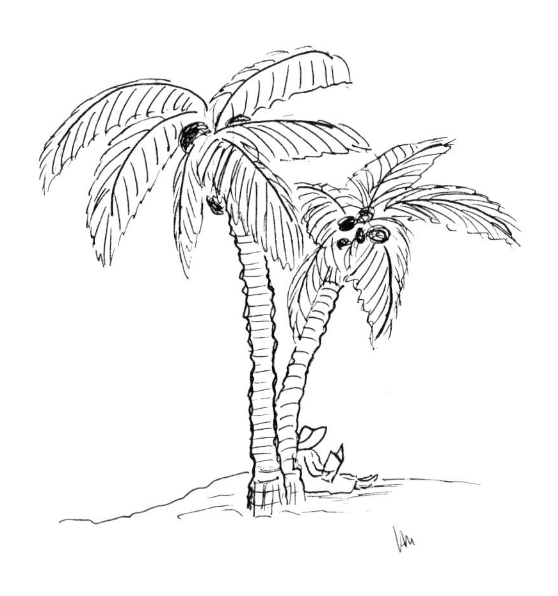

Adventure travel

The first all-woman expedition to Annapurna attracted the sexual attentions of the Sherpas, who inscribed large phalluses in the snow to enjoy vicarious pleasure from observation of the women's response. Women still risk stoning, imprisonment and expulsion in parts of Africa when they offend local traditions in dress or behaviour. Today, the emancipated woman, intent on going her own way, brushes aside the aggravating discomforts of travel; the fleas, bed-bugs and sweaty clothes, and endeavours to ignore petty, sexual prejudice and harassment. However, she should not ignore the health problems which can beset independent women travellers, destined for up-country adventure, and visits to third world nations. Long-haul flights, prolonged coach travel, high altitude, underwater swimming and solar irradiation can be particularly hazardous for women.

Menstrual problems

Some women on longer, hectic and strenuous journeys, stop menstruating which can be convenient but may be disquieting. This secondary amenorrhoea is probably associated, as in sportswomen, with intensive physical exercise and weight loss.

Travel can disturb the normal menstrual cycle. For their convenience and protection, many women travellers suppress ovulation and inhibit menstruation by taking oral contraceptive tablets on a continuous basis during the trip. An adequate supply of pills must be packed as they are not always available in developing countries or come unrecognisable as impregnated rice paper in places like China. Traveller's diarrhoea or motion sickness may disturb absorption, so protection may be lost. The need for antibiotics to treat infection may result in a similar problem of which the potential traveller should be made aware.

Case History 7.1

A young woman recently joined the practice list and requested an ante-natal clinic appointment. She had just spent a month in Borneo during which time she had suffered badly from gastro-enteritis with its associated diarrhoea and vomiting.

To her dismay on return to the UK, she found herself pregnant despite complying with oral contraceptive pill-taking instructions. She complained bitterly about her former general practitioner's failure to advise her of the need for further contraceptive precautions in the event of her experiencing vomiting and fluid loss during her travels. The doctor had apparently organised a course of vaccinations for her but had failed to offer any travel counselling. She chose to carry her baby to term but other girls in a similar situation have demanded therapeutic abortion.

Altitude sickness is more likely to occur in women on 'the pill' and those on oral contraceptives often incur marked fluid retention in the tropics.

Women who suffer from the premenstrual syndrome and menorrhagia have to consider how incapacitating the symptoms may be, added to the hassle and fatigue of modern travel. Tampons and sanitary towels are unobtainable in parts of Africa, Asia and South America, and they are scarce luxuries in many of the cities of the Russian Federation and former Eastern bloc countries. Changes in circadian rhythm with time-zone crossing on east/west long-haul flights can be a double-edged misery for women who can suffer from menstrual and urinary problems with enforced time-changes.

Urinary tract infections

Prolonged flying or coach journeys put the female bladder under considerable stress with resultant urological complaints. The absence or inadequacy of toilet facilities, a common phenomenon in world travel, can add to female difficulties. Fastidious western women are often psychologically unprepared to squat over a hole in the floor, bereft of washing facilities. Inadequate skin cleansing, sweating and inappropriate clothing can encourage monilial infection in the woman voyager and nether garments of open weave and natural fibre should be worn to reduce the risk of infection. Lower urinary tract infections (UTI) are commonplace in young women on foreign travel. The symptoms of cystitis can be disabling and there is always the risk of ascending pyelonephritis. Severe haematuria may occur and result in admission to a local clinic or hospital with facilities far below those of the West. Intravenous therapy or transfusion in many of these units carries the risk of AIDS transmission. Women, subject to recurrent UTI, should be advised to take an antibiotic excreted in the urine as a prophylactic during travel, to drink much fluid and to avoid alcohol.

Case History 7.2

On a recent teenage expedition to drought-ridden Zimbabwe, water was scarce for drinking and often unavailable for toilet purposes. Medicated wipes were unobtainable in the bush and the few remaining pools which had not dried up were infected with bilharzia. Eighteen percent of the girls in the party required treatment for urinary and vaginal infections. Poor fluid input and poor sanitary conditions led to a high incidence of infection.

Baring the nether regions in an inhospitable milieu can be hazardous. Advice from the female Annapurna team was 'if you must squat, squat high', otherwise leeches will attach themselves to exposed buttocks. In the Australian outback the advice is 'beware of the red-backed spider's bite on an exposed bottom' as it can have serious consequences. The necessary exposure of the rear for toilet purposes at high altitude risks frost bite and the problem is intensified if there is forced diuresis in women taking acetazolamide as a prophylactic against acute mountain sickness.

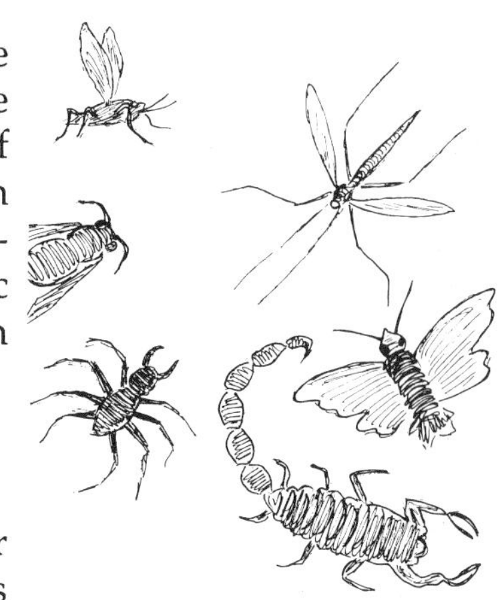

Vector-borne disease

Peripheral oedema

Girls on 'the pill' and older women with a poor venous circulation often accumulate peripheral oedema on long flights and coach tours. The resultant swollen ankles may be difficult to correct after the trip and the woman will, thereafter, suffer from a measure of stasis oedema. Elevation of the legs whenever possible and leg exercises on long journeys should be recommended. This will also diminish the risk of development of deep venous thrombosis and possible pulmonary embolism, which can afflict those taking hormonal contraception when undertaking prolonged journeys by air and coach. The associated relative immobility can be obstetrically dangerous.

Many girls indulge in sports activities on foreign tours and are exposed to hazards which do not affect their male companions. Women suffering significant PMS and menstrual symptoms should not undertake scuba-diving as severe cramps can mimic the signs of compression sickness. Menstruation is not, however, a contraindication to involvement in sub-aqua sporting activities. Menstrual blood loss need not attract the attention of sea predators but it is believed to attract bears. Menstrual blood absorbed by a tampon will not attract sharks. A tampon-protected swimmer in a jungle lagoon will not entice that other voracious water predator, the prihana. Female water skiers, however, risk foreign body penetration of the vagina and the inrush of contaminated water can result in ascending vaginal infections.

Travel and vacation encourage casual relationships and the risk of venereal and HIV infection. Condoms are not easily obtainable in many parts of the world and the woman traveller might be wise to carry them in anticipation of need. The marketing of Femidom, the female condom, now offers women the opportunity to ensure their own mechanical protection from potential sexually transmitted disease. Over-indulgence in cheap local alcohol can lower inhibitions and lead to coitus and genital infection.

Soft skin and bare legs are a target for mosquitoes, tsetse flies, ticks, leeches and sand-flies. Footwear should be worn on beaches and unprotected legs sprayed with insect repellants and covered on safari and in the evenings. Hair sprays, deodorants and cosmetics seem to attract biting insects and the wiser woman will limit their use during travel. Drug prophylaxis alone, will not ensure protection from malaria. Mechanical protection is very important. Bare shoulders and uncovered legs should be covered one hour before sunset in countries with a malarial risk. The female mosquito is at its most aggressive early and late in the day. Short skimpy dresses should be replaced by trousers for those intent on dawn and dusk animal safaris.

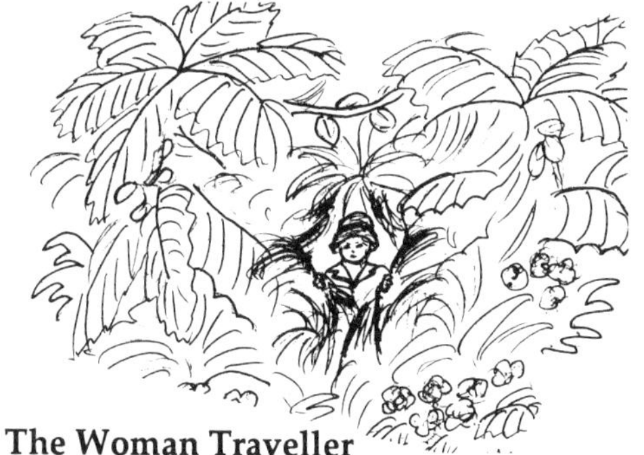

The Woman Traveller

Over-exposure to UVL puts the fair-skinned, blue-eyed blonde and the bikini-clad sun-worshipper at risk of neoplastic skin change. Sun avoidance and the use of sun-block preparations are now recommended. High factor sun-blocks – 15 and upwards – are required as a barrier to harmful ultra violet light absorption. Many women forget that actinic rays pass through thin blouses, through water and are particularly intense at high altitude. Sunlight over-exposure before 20 years of age, is more strongly associated with melanoma than after 30 years, especially if a blistering burn develops (Maducdoc 1992).

Phobias

Many women will be travelling abroad for the first time and some are inveigled into foreign holidays despite their apprehension about air travel. Travel phobias are common in women. A random sample study in my practice, showed that 16 percent of the cohort admitted to some phobia. Thirteen percent reported fear of flying with a female to male preponderance of 2:1 (McIntosh 1980). Anxiolytics, such as diazepam, should not be used in treatment but a beta-blocker may be of value in controlling palpitations. Behaviour-modification techniques are effective in dealing with this condition and desensitisation can be curative if there is time for treatment prior to travel.

Vehicular accident is the most likely hazard to befall the traveller and seat belt wear diminishes the fatalities but can cause breast trauma, lactiferous duct avulsion and haematomata. Nevertheless, the use of belts has to be encouraged even for the pregnant car passenger and despite the discomfort.

Pregnancy

Pregnant women travellers are not always aware of the limitations of travel insurance which may not cover premature labour or delivery abroad. The main danger is premature delivery where medical facilities are limited. Spontaneous abortions are more likely in smokers.

Case History 7.3

On an up-country trip to East Africa I was called one night to a nearby clinic to assist a woman in delayed second stage of labour. She had to be examined by candlelight. There were no mechanical delivery aids available and equipment had to be sterilised in a steel flask heated over an open outside wood fire.

The toilet block was separated from the unit and was fifty yards away. The nearest back-up medical facility was two hours away by dirt track. The decrepit ambulance pressed into service to make this journey had never been known to make the intervening distance without mechanical breakdown. Fortunately, mother and baby made the journey successfully and the baby was delivered by ventouse extraction.

Commercial air travel is not hazardous to mother or fetus. Flying in pressurised aircraft is allowed by most

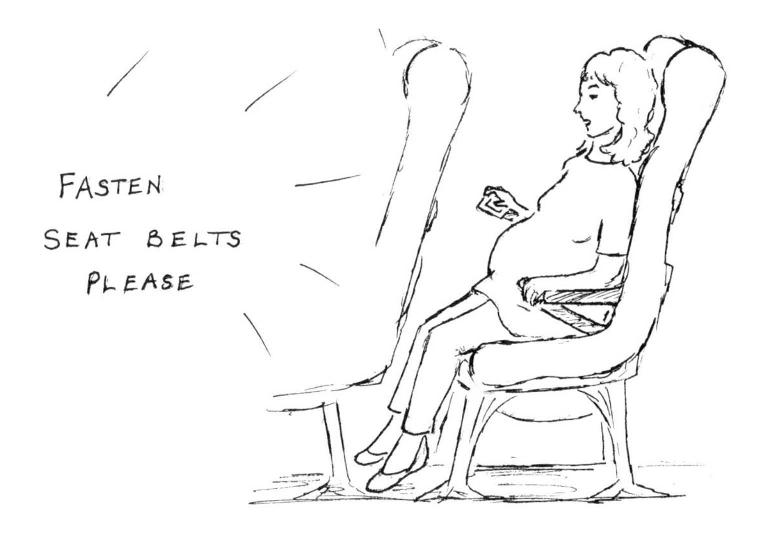

Figure 7.1: The Pregnant Traveller

companies up to 35 weeks of pregnancy with a doctor's note confirming the expected date of delivery. Commercial jets maintain the cabin pressure at about 5000 to 8000 feet above sea level. If a woman suffers from a condition which interferes with uteroplacental blood flow such as anaemia or toxaemia, or with placental integrity such as placental separation, even such a relatively small drop in the oxygen partial pressure may adversely affect the fetus and air travel is not advised.

Travel in any vehicle – plane, bus or train and sitting in cramped positions for long periods will result in increased dependent oedema, low back and pubic symphysis discomfort, calf muscle cramps and the risk of superficial and deep venous thrombosis. Pregnant women should be encouraged to use aisle seats, walk for about 15 minutes every hour, find ways to prop up their legs and stretch their backs. Seat belts should be worn low across the pubis and below the anterior iliac spine. On planes in the later stages of pregnancy, they should avoid greasy foods and gassy drinks as flatulence is increased at altitude.

Holidaying at high altitude over seven thousand feet should be avoided as there is evidence that intrauterine growth can be retarded, the birth weight being inversely related to altitude at each gestational age beyond 35 weeks and it is possible that high altitude trekking may create problems for the fetus.

While swimming is excellent exercise, water skiing and water chutes can be hazardous, and serious but rare vulval and vaginal lacerations, and even traumatic peritonitis have been reported.

The onset of premature labour or threatened abortion in a woman travelling through a developing country can be highly dangerous for mother and baby. Medical facilities may be many miles or hours away; if present, they may be grossly inadequate and even insanitary; immediacy of medical aid is unlikely and although local midwives may be capable they will often lack appropriate equipment. There may be a lack of piped water, no disposables, no delivery assisting appliances, infusion fluid and blood transfusion, if available, may be contaminated and harbour HIV infection.

Pregnant travellers are at special risk of deep venous thrombosis (DVT) on long-haul flights and protracted coach journeys, and should exercise at 45 minute intervals if at all possible, during travel. Increased coagulability, compression of the venacava by the gravid uterus, venous dilation and immobility are a dangerous combination and the risk of DVT is increased five fold during pregnancy (Nicholson 1992). Scuba diving should be avoided as appropriate depth/time diving cannot be established for the pregnant, and recompression procedures can damage the foetus.

Pregnant women are susceptible to listeriosis and should avoid cook/chill meals, paté and soft cheeses abroad, as these may be contaminated.

Table 7.1 Advice for Pregnant Travellers

Avoid live vaccination if at all possible, and certainly during the first trimester

Assume air travel will not be possible after 35th week of gestation

Avoid travel to countries where there is resistance to conventional malaria therapy

Consider availability of medical aid and quality of facilities, and speed of evacuation to the UK in countries to be visited

Avoid residence at areas above 7,000 ft altitude

Be aware of the dangers of hepatitis and HIV infection from infected needles and transfusion equipment in the majority of third world countries and in up-country situations

When complicating medical and obstetric conditions are known to exist, a journey to an undeveloped nation or up-country area may be contraindicated. Some countries refuse to admit women in the later stages of pregnancy and insurance protection may not cover delivery abroad and/or exclude medical care for premature labour or hospitalisation.

Vaccination prophylaxis and pregnancy

Live vaccinations should not be given in pregnancy if practicable and should certainly be avoided in the first trimester. Inactivated polio vaccine can be given and tetanus vaccination of the mother will give protection to the baby in the neonatal period. Hepatitis A infection is more severe in pregnancy and immunoglobulin cover can be given to those likely to be at risk. Enteric-transmitted non-A non-B hepatitis has a ten percent fatality rate in the pregnant and immunoglobulin is not of proven efficacy. Vaccines which can be given with caution if really necessary are rabies, diphtheria, tetanus and meningococcal polysaccharide. The effect of new vaccines for hepatitis A and B on fetal development remains to be assessed. Neither is currently recommended in pregnancy unless there is a definite risk of hepatitis infection while the patient is abroad. If pregnant women have to travel through infected areas of India, Asia and Africa they must scrupulously avoid possibly contaminated water and food.

Table 7.2: Information for Pregnant Travellers

On long journeys:

- Use aisle seats in aircraft
- Walk about for 15 minutes in every hour
- Find means of propping up the legs and stretching the back
- Wear seat belt low across the pubis and below ant. iliac spines
- Avoid aerated drinks and alcohol

Malaria complications are more common in pregnancy and prophylaxis is vital. Chloroqine is a safe prophylactic and proguanil, an anti-folate, should be given with a folic acid supplement. The pregnant should avoid travel to countries where there is resistance to conventional antimalarial therapy.

Table 7.3 Medical management of the pregnant traveller

- Avoid vaccination in the first trimester and if possible thereafter
- Discourage visits to countries where there is resistance to conventional malaria prophylaxis
- consider the need for folic acid supplementation in patients taking antimalarials.
- Avoid prescribing primaquin as there is risk of glucose-6-dehydrogenase deficiency in the foetus. Mefloquin is contraindicated
- Advise on the risks of peripheral oedema and venous thrombosis and pulmonary embolism with prolonged sitting
- Warn of the dangers of dehydration if the patient contracts travellers' diarrhoea

Today, women travellers will not be deflected from travel to the most remote parts of the globe and exploration of the world's high places and ocean depths. An awareness of special medical risks, suitable precautions and prophylaxis will ensure that most will travel in relative safety. Wise pre-travel counselling from and informed doctor or nurse will help them to reach new objectives in good health.

References

Banerjee A (1989). Belts and breasts, *Travel Med Intl*, **7:3**, 132.
Barry M (1989). Pregnancy and travel, *J Amer Med Assoc*, **261**, 728–731.
Dembert M (1987). Health advice for the travelling scuba diver, *Travel Med Intl*, **5:2**, 61–64.
Dembert M (1986). Health advice for the woman traveller, *Travel Med Intl*, **4:4**, 175–179.

Kirby R (1990). Urological complaints during travel, *Travel Med Intl*, **8:3**, 104–105.
Macducdol L, Wagner R *et al* (1992). *Archives of Dermatology*, **128**, 628-629.
McIntosh I B (1990). The stress of modern travel, *Travel Med Intl*, **8:3**, 118–121.
McIntosh I B (1980). Incidence, management and treatment of phobias, *Pharm Med*, **1:2**, 77–82.
Nicholson P J (1992). Pregnancy and Vacational Flying, *Travel Med Internl*, **10.3**, 105-108.
Robinson J (1990). *Wayward women. A guide to the female* traveller, Oxford University Press.
Russell M (1986). *Blessings of a good thick skirt*, Collins.
Walker E and Williams G (1983). ABC of travel, *Br Med J*, **286**, 1339.

CHAPTER 8

THE ELDERLY TRAVELLER

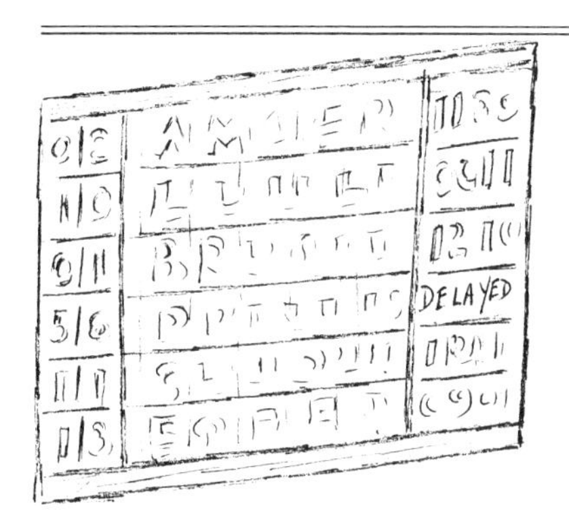

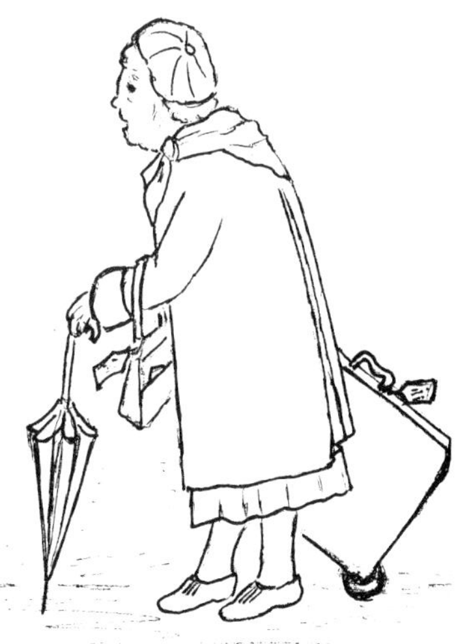

Figure 8.1: The Elderly Traveller

Summary

The number of elderly people in the developed nations of the world is surging ahead, and those over 75 years of age in Britain will make up 22 percent of the population by the end of the century. Of these, 80 percent are known to be able to travel from their homes with little assistance (MacLennon W 1988) and many are embarking on extensive travel by road, sea and air. With the anticipated expansion of global travel, a rise in the numbers of aged voyagers is inevitable and health risks will rise accordingly.

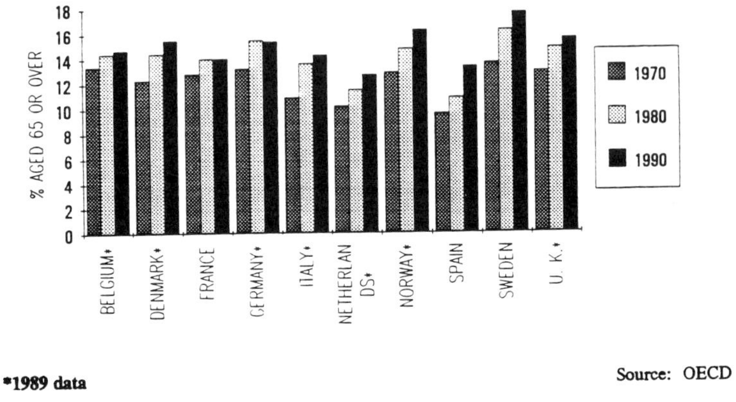

Figure 8.2: Proportion of population aged 65 or over

Affluent senior citizens, freed from the constraints of work, family and time, are enthusiastically grasping opportunities for world exploration, often with scant regard for their well-being in foreign climes and hostile environments. The potential reduction in travel time and fatigue, linked with special facilities, make air travel a favoured mode of transport for those of advanced years. Fortunately, few patients are medically unacceptable as air passengers.

Facts and figures

In a 25 percent quota sample, a survey of over 65 year old travellers in my practice (McIntosh 1991) showed that more than a third of the cohort had travelled outwith the UK in the last year and 41.7 percent in the previous three years. A remarkable 30.8 percent of over 80 year olds had also travelled abroad within three years. Of all travellers,

80.8 percent travelled by air and 9.5 percent by sea with others using varying modes of transport.

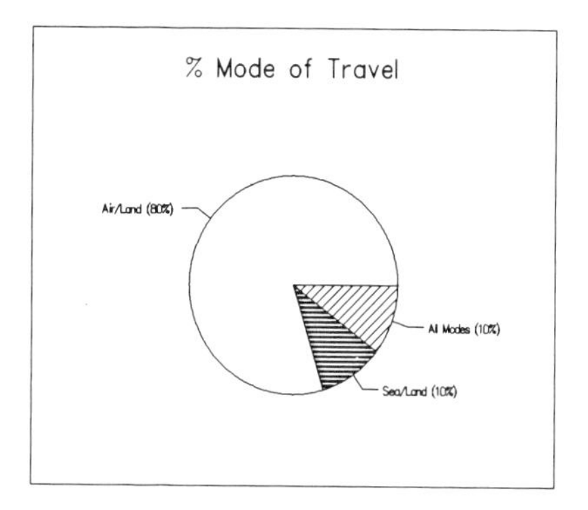

Figure 8.3: Mode of travel

The majority travelled to Europe and Africa with the third largest group to the USA.

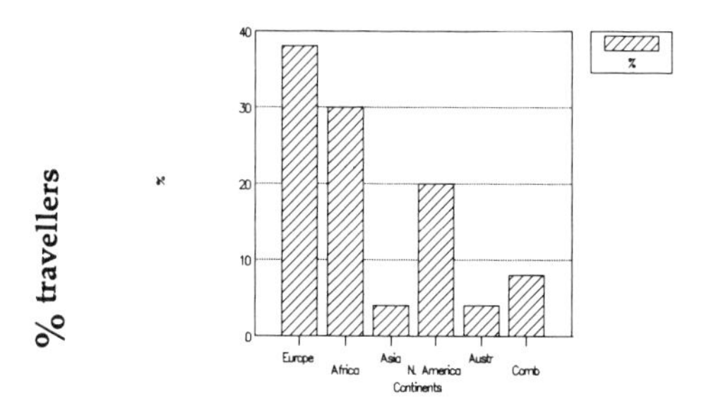

Figure 8.4: Destinations - % Continents Visited

While abroad, 45 percent of the travellers became ill, 59 percent of those becoming ill at their destination. There was no serious imported infectious disease. Of the European travellers, 56 percent became ill with 32 percent of them affected by diarrhoea and vomiting. In those visiting Africa 45 percent succumbed, with 14 percent suffering from enteritis. Although the number was small, all those visiting Asia also contracted intestinal disorder. Significantly fewer travellers to North America became ill (24 percent). Of all illnesses, 53 percent were gastrointestinal, second place being occupied with cardiovascular events in much lower incidence; 18 percent required consultation with a doctor abroad; 58 percent sought the immediate attention of the family doctor on return from holiday and 18 percent of ill travellers were admitted to hospital outwith Britain. In several cases, insurance cover excluded pre-existing disease: 30 percent of the tourists had travelled alone with 35 percent of this number becoming ill, thus adding to the psychological distress associated with the physical illness.

Case history 8.1

One patient reported travelling without insurance. She was admitted to an American hospital with gall-bladder disease and was presented with a large bill for professional health services. She had travelled regularly for many years without travel insurance cover, However, this single hospital admission was so costly she could not afford to travel to the USA again.

These findings suggest that older travellers may be at higher risk from travel-contracted disease. The high proportion of European and African travellers probably reflects the high number of package tours to the Mediterranean littoral where Cossar *et al* have reported a very high incidence of gastro-enteritis.

The high percentage of returning travellers requiring GP assistance draws attention to the impact of travel-induced illness on primary care resources. The number of hospital admissions abroad suggests illness of a serious nature and the considerable number becoming ill when travelling alone, and sometimes without insurance, must cause concern.

Air travel

Cabin pressures equivalent to 5000-8000 feet create the physiological hazard of hypoxia for older travellers and place at risk those with little cardiac, cerebrovascular, respiratory and haematological reserve (Chapman *et al*, 1988). The risk can, however, be diminished by the judicious use of in-flight oxygen. The expansion of gases trapped in body cavities such as the sinuses and the bowel also creates a problem but absolute contra-indications to air travel are few. Difficulties can often be resolved by a week or two of delay in planned transportation.

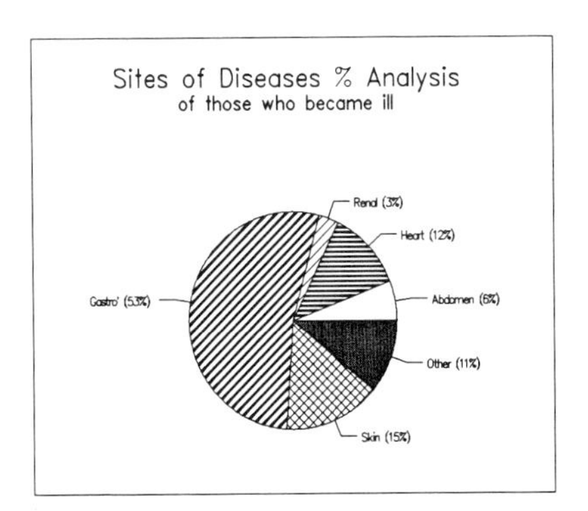

Figure 8.5: Effects of travel on the older traveller

Excluded passengers

Patients with severe anaemia, very recent myocardial infarction, cerebrovascular acccident, gastrointestinal haemorrhage, or major chest or abdominal surgery, and those with uncontrolled, congestive cardiac failure will be denied carriage. The unescorted, confused elderly, agitated dements and the psychotic are also refused passage for obvious reasons of airline safety.

Table 8.2: Excluded passengers: those with -

— severe anaemia
— very recent myocardial infarction
— cerebrovascular accident
— gastrointestinal haemorrhage
— major chest or abdominal surgery
— uncontrolled congestive cardiac failure
— unescorted confused elderly
— agitated dements
— psychotic

Between 1977 and 1984 IATA reported 577 deaths in the air, 326 of which had cardiac causation and 56 had prior medical problems. A total of 247 were given assistance by an on-board physician.

Companies are, of course, dependent on potential passengers revealing their current state of health at the time of booking and many prospective clients, intent on travel to loved ones or specialist clinics, choose to conceal medical frailties and disabilities. Leading airlines require booking agents to obtain a standardised medical information form from such passengers with a special version for the use of the disabled who travel frequently. The passenger's family doctor is then approached for details of the patient's current medical state and special requirements. This information identifies those at special risk and ensures provision of wheelchairs, special seating, diets, supplementary oxygen and transit assistance for those in need.

Easing the burden

The trauma of travel can be minimised for every elderly traveller by intelligent anticipation of need. Wheelchair or buggy travel can eliminate the physical demands involved in negotiation of long corridors and arrival halls. Special lifting arrangements remove the need for climbing steps and gangways. Boeing 747 and Tristar aircraft now carry on-board wheelchairs. The 'skychair' designed specifically for in-flight use provides easy transport to cabin toilets.

Pre-planning and early booking can ensure that cabin seating for the infirm is obtained close to toilet accommodation, with priority given to proximity to the specially designated disabled persons' toilet available on most intercontinental flights. Old and infirm passengers can expect attendant help to reach the toilet but this assistance is denied within the confines of the toilet as flight stewards have food-handler status. Thus elderly and disabled air travellers must be capable of managing their own wheelchair transfer and intimate functions. Many of the old endeavour to avoid these problems by missing out their diuretic therapy on the day of travel and as a consequence often go into congestive cardic failure on long-haul flights. Unexpected stop-overs at remote staging posts may find inadequate toilet facilities to sustain the aged transit passenger.

Geriatric patients frequently forget to carry regular medication within hand luggage with consequent panic requests en route for drugs vital to well-being. Many fail to appreciate that they can be divorced from baggage by misrouting, handlers' strikes or suddenly altered flight arrangements due to bad weather or technical failure.

Case history 2

One elderly woman left home at 6 a.m. to make a visit to relatives in Canada, having carefully chosen a 10 a.m. non-stop flight to ensure reaching her destination on the east coast in the shortest time possible in daylight hours. On reaching Prestwick she found her plane had an engine fault. The initial anticipated three-hour delay extended first to six hours and then to nine. During most of the intervening hours she sat patiently in the departure lounge and by the flight departure her legs were swollen to the knees. A lightning air-controllers' strike occurred when the aircraft was over the Atlantic and it was diverted to Detroit. After a night arrival, she was transferred to a coach for the long journey to Toronto. By dawn the poor woman had been travelling and sitting for 24 hours, had become increasingly breathless, with legs swollen to mid-thigh. Her shoes were almost enveloped by the overhanging oedema at the ankles.

She went into congestive cardiac failure shortly after crossing the Canadian border and was taken from the bus to hospital to be left in the hands of strangers many miles from her destination and a long-waiting, distraught daughter. Most of her holiday was spent in hospital and in convalescence. She returned home much the worse for her protracted air journey. Her cardiac failure is now controlled but prolonged engorgement and distension has ruined her peripheral venous system, and she suffers chronic postural oedema. She is now vehement that she will make no more Atlantic crossings.

British Airways offers Travelwise advice leaflets to elderly and incapacitated passengers giving sensible instructions on how they can ameliorate the rigours of the long seat-bound hours of flight.

In-flight immobility

Many of the aged rarely leave the security of their seats while on board. Movement on long flight sectors would diminish the gross peripheral oedema suffered by many senior passengers in prolonged travel. The risks of deep venous thrombosis and pulmonary embolism have been high-lighted (Cruikshank *et al*, 1988). Peripheral superficial femoral arterial vessel occlusion in association with long-haul flying has also been reported (Teenan, 1992) and orthostatic purpura of the lower limbs (Bourke 1992) in older individuals with no previous history of peripheral vascular disease. Immobility and dehydration appear to be factors contributing to arterial occlusion on long-haul flights. There is a case for the very old to take an aspirin tablet before subjecting themselves to long exposure to restrictive seating by air or land. Regular movement of foot and leg muscles while seated should become standard advice to all such passengers. The old should be encouraged to mobilise and exercise limbs at transit stops. Many choose to remain seated within the cabin, and are often encouraged to do so by staff for reasons of management convenience. These strictures also apply to those on coaches, for long land tours attract a preponderance of elderly passengers.

Other ill-effects

Changes in environment, altitude effects and disturbance to circadian rhythm can upset the mildly confused patient and precipitate crisis in aged demented patients.

The elderly diabetic

It is probably wiser for diabetics tablet medication or dietary restriction to follow the time operative at point of departure until arrival at destination, rather than changing the hours with the crossing of time zones. They then can take meals and medication close to their normal pattern.

The old diabetic on insulin can be deleteriously affected by crossing time zones, unaccustomed exercise, altered diet management and anxiety. An increase or decrease of 2-4 percent of daily insulin per hour of time shift is advised for the insulin dependent, determined by direction of travel and length of the flight (see Figure 8.4). The British diabetic Association offers travel guides for diabetics, covering 70 destinations (see Appendix). The diabetic, those on H_2 antagonists and diuretics and the 60 percent of those over 60 years with achlorhydria are at special risk from that scourge of travellers, diarrhoea. Inadequate toilet facilities at transit airports can be disastrous for the old with precarious bladder control, especially if they have a functional disability.

Senescent and arthritic patients with stiff hips or fixed knees are at particular disadvantage within the narrow confines of aircraft and coaches. They benefit from judicious use of aisle seating away from bulkheads. A placement in the extended space by emergency exits seems attractive, but many companies operate a covert policy excluding the disabled from such seats as they might obstruct evacuation.

Inadequate medical care

The promotion of adventurous world travel rarely precludes the old, and one meets septa- and octagenerians on the grand tour of China, taking in the delights of Lake Titicaca, sampling Amazonia or tackling, despite hip replacements, minor peaks in the Himalayas. They do so, protected by the apparent security of world-wide insurance cover, forgetting that initial medical aid will come from the local clinic or hospital. This may be able to offer only minor first aid and have few facilities. The poor quality of immediate care cannot be obviated. Many of the travelling aged, accustomed to prompt and appropriate medical attention, are unaware of the abyss of inadequate care which can befall them if they wander through the more adventurous paths of world tourism. Even popular

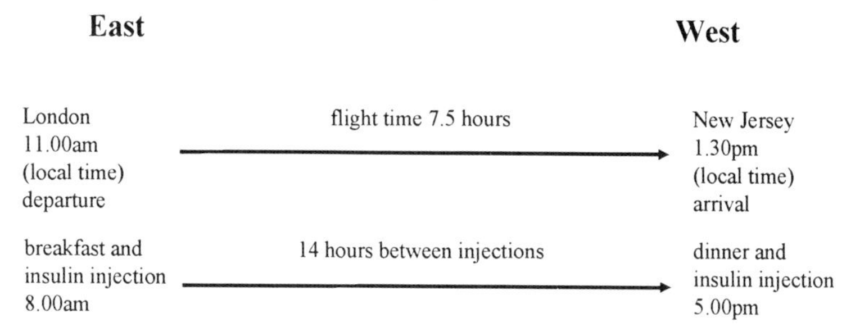

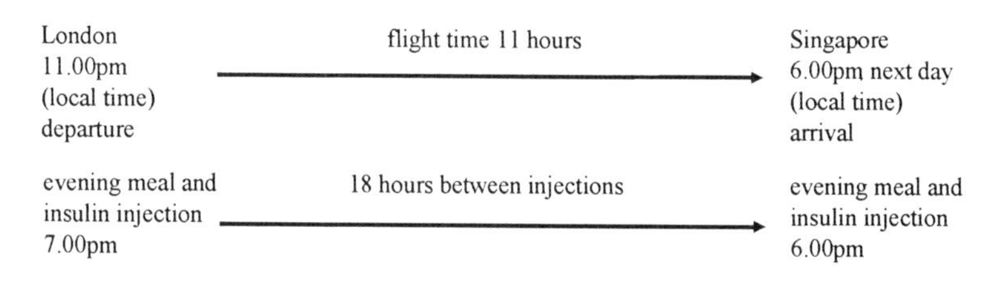

Figure 8.6: Time zone crossing and insulin dosage

vacation resorts may reveal a standard far below that required by a geriatric presenting with multi system disturbance as a result of dehydration, failed drug compliance or cardiac failure.

Extremes of altitude and temperature

Unsuspecting aged patients can expose themselves abruptly to the thin air of high altitude airports in their quest to follow the Incas to Machu Picchu in Peru or gain a sight of Everest from the hotel at Namche Bazaar, Nepal. Those with minimal cardiac reserve find themselves gasping with dyspnoea or wracked with angina from hypoxia. Cerebral arterial insufficiency may result in confusion, imbalance and the risk of fracture from falls. A 24-hour period of rest is mandatory for old folk arriving suddenly at high altitude.

The old are likely to suffer heat-stroke when visiting the Valley of the Kings at Luxor. They are also at high risk of transient ischaemic attacks and stroke when over-exposed to high temperatures. Dehydration from enteritis, the scourge of travel, can easily thrust the older voyager into fluid and metabolic imbalance in hot countries. High fluid input is essential for the ageing traveller with full electrolyte replacement.

Case history 3

Two of my elderly patients set off on a tour of Russian Central Asia. They suffered minor gastric upsets in Moscow and were physically ill-equipped to withstand the rigours of travel in Central Asia and Tadzikistan. Severe gastroenteritis struck in Tashkent and was followed promptly by dehydration and debility. Both had to be warded in an isolation unit in the local

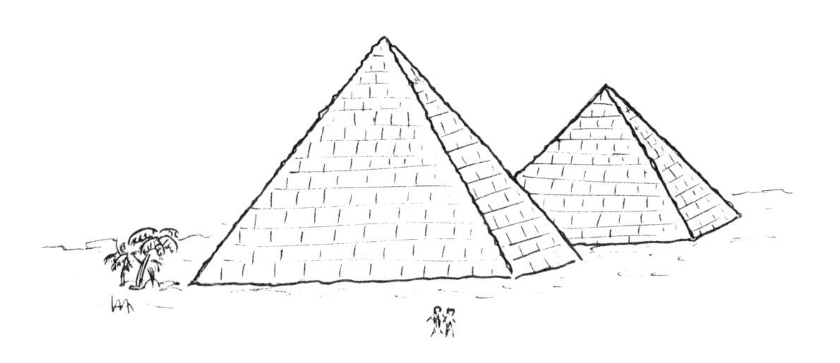

The 'Blue Rinse' adventure

infectious disease unit. Doctors and nurses were kind to them but facilities were limited, wards sparse and therapy draconian. Stripped naked, they were hosed down with tepid water by nursing aides before being bedded down in a cell-like ward, inside grounds with high walls and electronically-operated exits controlled by police. The husband returned home with a campylobacter infection which resisted therapy. He steadily lost weight, fell as a result of weakness, fractured his pelvis and never recovered.

Time-zone change

To avoid the deleterious effects of jet-lag, the old should consider 24 hours of rest after a five-hour time zone change.

Sun and sea

Old age pensioners benefit from the availability of a ship's medical officer and cruising holidays are popular with the old. An unstable environment with many gangways, wide stairways and long passage-ways increases the likelihood of falls and fractures. It exacerbates the poor balance which is a common feature of advanced years.

The ageing skin can suffer seriously from exposure to ultraviolet rays at altitude or from reflected light from snow or sea which can result in lesions of actinic keratosis or the activation of malignant change. The use of sun-blocks, head and face protection and avoidance of exposure to the direct tropical sun has to be recommended to the geriatric traveller.

Slow skin healing makes bites and puncture wounds potentially serious and vector-borne local infection should be avoided.

Case history 4

A 75-year-old patient returned from a month's ramble in Nepal and presented in the surgery complaining of an itch in two areas of his scalp which had been exposed to the sun. One lesion was an obvious area of actinic keratosis which only required a touch of liquid notrogen to put right. The other was a lentigo maligna and was removed with minor surgery. With a slightly apologetic 'while I'm here Doc' comment, he drew attention to a small, flat brown nodule on his lower thigh which had been exposed to sunlight when he was wearing shorts. He thought it had become bigger recently but had been aware of its presence over many years. It looked benign and was considered so by the

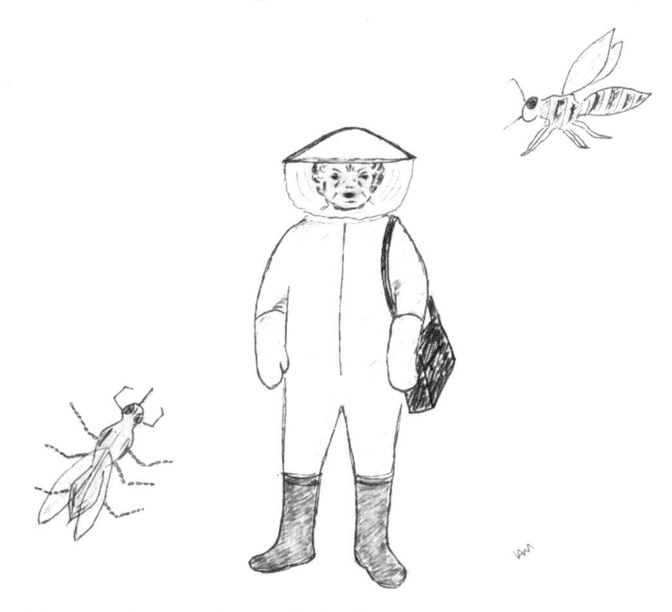

Avoidance of vector-borne infection

dermatologist but a biopsy confirmed malignant melanoma of 2mm penetration. More radical surgery was required in treatment. The effects of high altitude sunlight on his exposed skin were considered to be a contributory factor in his skin changes.

Senescence undoubtedly adds to the many problems facing those who cavort across the world, and the elderly traveller, or the carer, must anticipate potential difficulties of transport, transit and tour. Appraisal of risk and preplanning can maximise comfort and minimise hazard. Much depends upon experience, denied the first time traveller who may have recourse to books such as The Complete Traveller (Bakewell, 1977) or The Traveller's Handbook (Dawood, 1992), or depend upon travel agent or family doctor for timely advice.

The likely advent of non-stop flights to the Pacific and Australia and their use by many old and very old passengers, demands more information on airline and on-board facilities be made available. Airport altitudes, ambient temperatures and the adequacy of local medical services should be provided by the former. All airlines should consider the issue of instructive leaflets and in-flight videos to advise on methods of combating long-flight immobility in captive older passengers and might encourage staff to offer such advice.

Family doctors will increasingly be approached for travel recommendations and a reasoned response will depend on awareness of the risks and facilities. Good avice, careful consideration and sound pre-planning will ensure that the elderly are not denied their desire for cautious adventure and safe travel to the more accessible corners of our shrinking world.

Patient leaflets advising Dos and Don'ts for elderly travellers can augment verbal advice and counselling, eg:

Dos and Don'ts for the elderly traveller

DO:

— Plan ahead to obtain maximal airline assistance

— Take normal daily medication

— Take a supply of routine medication with the hand luggage

— Walk about within the aeroplane and exercise the legs

— Drink plenty of water or juice on the air journey

— Rest for 24 hours after a journey across time zones

— Treat water as suspect unless known to be uncontaminated

— Take up all appropriate vaccinations and prophylactics

— Purchase adequate health insurance

DO NOT:

— Drink alcohol on the flight

— Remain seat-bound for the whole flight

— Pack necessary medication in luggage bound for the hold

— Leave routine medication at home

— Assume that doctors and hospitals abroad provide as good a service as that normally experienced

— Drink water abroad unless it has been treated

Table 8.4: Air travel recommendations for the elderly

1 — Anticipate and prepare for medical problems
2 — Consider a medical check-up before departure
3 — Warn airline of special medical, dietary or mobility requirements
4 — Organise vaccination and prophylaxis
5 — continue routine medication en route and carry it in hand luggage
6 — Purchase adequate, inclusive medical insurance
7 — Exercise the legs whenever possible in flight
8 — Drink plenty of water and juices on board
9 — Avoid pulses, salads and alcohol with in-flight meals
10 — Rest up for 24 hours after arrival at destination

Table 8.5: Management of the elderly traveller

1 — Clinically examine high risk patients
2 — Review routine drug therapy
3 — Advise need for special adjustments to in-flight therapy, eg. insulin
4 — Organise appropriate vaccinations and prophylaxis
5 — Stress need to carry and maintain medication en route
6 — Advise patient to report invalid status to the airline
7 — Council on special risks of altitude, extremes of heat and cold, immobility, cabin air pressure and humidity, jet-lag and effects of environmental disturbance
8 — Stress need for adequate, inclusive holiday medical insurance cover

Table 8.6: Instruction sheet for the diabetic traveller

1 — Find out flight times, duration and departure/arrival in local time

2 — Remember to carry in the hand-luggage insulin, syringes, tablets, blood glucose strips (three times the amount for the time away

3 — Take a supply of glucose tablets

4 — Travel-sickness can upset the dosage routine

5 — Monitor blood sugar levels before and after a flight and two or three times on the plane if a long journey

6 — Time zone adjustments may be necessary

7 — Running levels a bit 'high' for 24 hours of travel is unlikely to do any harm

8 — If unexpected delay occurs extending interval between injections for more than 15 hours, take an extra small dose of insulin with food.

9 — Take extra care of the feet if the holiday involves much waling in very hot/cold or humid conditions, or prolonged sitting in transport vehicles

10 — Check holiday insurance covers diabetes

References

Bakewell J (1977). *The Complete Traveller*, 246-248, Sidgewick & Jackson

Bourke J P (1992) Intercontinental flights and orthostatic purpura, *Br Med J*, **305**, 1588.

Chapman P *et al* (1988). *J Amer Med Assoc*, **259**, 1983-1988

Cossar J H, Reid D, Fellon R J *et al* (1990). A cummulative review of studies on travellers, *J Infect*, **21**, 27-42

Cruikshank J M *et al* (1988). *The Lancet*, **ii**, 497-498

Dawood R (1992). *How to stay healthy abroad*, 2nd ed, Oxford University Press

Editorial (1985). *The Lancet*, **i**, 28-29

Joseph M (1977). *The Businessman's Travel Handbook*, Paddington Press

MacLennan W J (1988). The ageing society, *Br J Hosp* Med, **39,** 112-120
McIntosh I (1991). Travel Induced Illness: a GP based survey, *Scot Med*, **11.4**, 14-15.
Mills F J *et al* (1983). Medical emergencies in the air II: Equipment and prevention, *Br Med J*, **286**, 1204-1206
Teenan R P *et al* (1992). Peripheral arterial thrombosis related to commercial airline flights, *Br J Clin Pract*, **46:3**, 165-166
Wakeford R (1986). Death in the clouds, *Br Med J*, **293**, 1642-1643

Useful Address

Diabetes Care Dept, British Diabetic Association, 10 Queen Street London W1M 0BD

CHAPTER 9

THE DISABLED AND HANDI-CAPPED TRAVELLER

Determined, goal-orientated disabled people can and do make remarkable world trips and adventurous undertakings. In return for a little extra health risk, their travels can bring rich individual reward. The travel industry is slowly endeavouring to accommodate the needs of the less than physically perfect and their incapacity should not preclude desired international travel. Travel health clinics can identify their special needs and doctors and nurses should be able to offer them sound counsel.

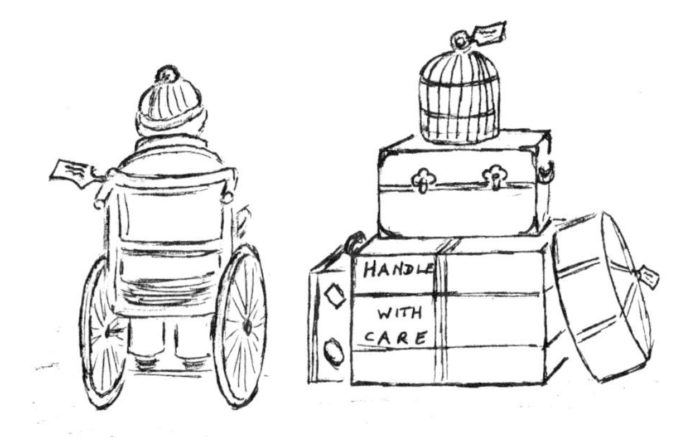

Figure 9.1: The Disabled Traveller

Although global travels may be possible, they undoubtedly face problems and hostility which are spared their healthier companions and many parts of the world are quite inappropriate destinations. Well-developed countries are, however, becoming better prepared to provide the extra services required by the handicapped. A change in attitude in some populations with regard to the physically underprivileged has seen a move away from entrenched antagonism.

There are three million disabled people in the UK under the age of 75. Despite their physical and mental incapacity, many wish to travel. Physical handicap is not an insurmountable barrier to international journeying. The need for cautious anticipatory travel planning and medical assessment is, however, a vital pre-requisite if these travellers are to relocate in safety. Proposed route, transport mode and destination are major considerations in determining the additional hazards of travel for the less able and their need for additional support. A lack or absence of facilities for the physically disadvantaged is the norm in third world and impoverished countries, and over much of Eastern Europe and Asia. Some societies are psychologically unprepared to recognise their special needs and may even positively discriminate against them.

Excluding minor physical impairment, individuals suffering severe physical frailty, functional disability and handicap are best advised to restrict foreign travel to countries best equipped to accommodate their needs. These are listed in Table 9.1.

Table 9.1: Countries best equipped to deal with disabled travellers

United Kingdom and Ireland
Scandinavia
Northern Europe
Republic of South Africa
New Zealand
Australia
Hong Kong and Singapore
North America including the United States of America and Canada

This does not mean that these countries present no problems for disabled travellers but there is State recognition of the need to provide for those unfortunate enough to suffer degrees of physical inadequacy. Psychologically too, the population of these countries are likely to react more positively in support of individuals with such limitations.

In some advanced countries, however, antidiscrimination laws may even work against the provision of special services which publicly identify those with infirmity. They cannot, for instance, be specifically named in broadcast calls for early aeroplane boarding in the United States. Unknown environments full of potential hazard can intimidate the handicapped. Transit through airports, train and bus stations and by plane, ship and train can be a challenge and a threat to the disabled traveller in terms of access and possible health risk.

The caring family doctor or the nurse or physician consulting in the travel clinic should be prepared to tailor advice to those with different categories of disability. For assessment purposes, categories of physical malfunction can be divided into the visible, the invisible, the ambulatory and non-ambulatory, the stable and the non-static. Visible conditions may attract more attention and possibly more proffered assistance whereas the invisible may be less embarrassing but will not generate unsolicited support

Table 9.2: Categories of handicap

Categories of handicap
The invisible, eg deafness, poor sight
The visible
The ambulatory
The non-ambulatory
The stable
The non-static

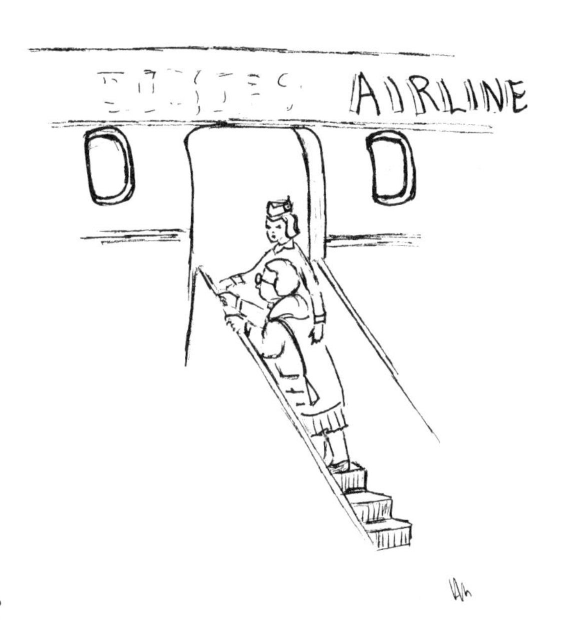

Fit to travel?

Air travel

Enforced immobility in disabled travellers may well increase the risk of deep venous thrombosis formation and pulmonary embolism on long-haul flights and they should be encouraged to exercise the limbs and flex and extend limb muscles as frequently as possible during the journey.

Those with spastic and arthritic limbs meet similar problems in air travel. Inability to stretch and move limbs brings cramp and the risk of thrombosis formation and pulmonary embolism. The affluent should be encouraged to travel executive or club class to win extra leg room.

IATA, the International Air Travel Transport Association has produced the MEDIF and FREMEC cards to be completed by disabled potential passengers. Part 1 of the MEDIF is completed by the passenger and Part 2 by the passenger's doctor. Provision of this information depends on the patient's willingness to comply and the accuracy in completion of the health statement.

Many incapacitated individuals still present to airlines without having completed these forms and airline agents can refuse onward transportation. Prior notification of physical incapacity is essential to ensure appropriate support on the day of transportation and transit.

Blind travellers

Guide dogs cannot accompany blind passengers on external flights across borders without the dog undergoing unrealistically lengthy quarantine which is impractical for the blind vacationer. Blind passengers using canes are usually allowed to retain them by their seat in the aircraft but stringent application of security rules may mean that over-zealous authorities will forbid them in the cabin. However, stewardesses will normally guide passengers to seating and the toilets.

Hotels and restaurants, airlines and transport systems provide few other additional facilities for the blind. Few boarding instructions are provided in braille and many airports and an increasing number of railway stations now only provide departure information visually or inaudibly on a public address system. Safe travel for the blind usually dictates the need for travel with a sighted companion. BA in association with the Royal Society for the Blind produce a useful tape for blind air passengers.

Limb deformities

Limb angulations, fixed limbs, joint replacement and arthritis may restrict access to trains, planes and coaches, and the confined space of long-haul flights may create severe cramps and spasms in the afflicted.

Management

Cautious prescribing of Diazepam or Dantrolene for prolonged flights may decrease pain from spasm. Loss of joint mobility makes for difficulty in accommodating limbs in the narrow confines of the aircraft cabin. Passengers should be advised to pre-book aircraft seating and take advantage of seat positions with additional leg space. They should avoid seating next to the body of the aircraft, facing bulkheads and where it is impossible to recline seats. The incapacitated passenger should seek an aisle seat as this permits extension of at least one limb into the passageway and eases exit for exercise and toilet purposes.

Locomotor problems with imbalance and disabled limbs do create difficulties on stairs, long walkways, lurching companionway and decks with a very real risk of falls and fracture.

Wheelchair-bound travellers

The wheelchair-bound passenger may face access problems on aeroplanes, trains and buses. Appropriate rampage, wheelchair access and disabled transport is available at major international airports but in smaller airports and in transit situations these may be inadequate or non-existent. Newer, wide-bodied aeroplanes such as the Boeing 747 and the newest DC 10s carry onboard wheelchairs but the disabled traveller should ideally travel with his or her own lightweight folding wheelchair.

Travel health consultants should advise on potential problems of ramp and lift facilities within the airport, on the air-side and in the aircraft. The size of the aircraft, rampage, wheelchair carriage and lavatory access are all relevant details. Transit points must be carefully considered. In many parts of the Middle East and Asia used in transit or stopovers on long-haul flights, provisions for the frail and disabled are often inadequate. It has to be ensured that at no point in a multi-leg journey, will a small plane be used for a shuttle or feeder service.

Table 9.3: Air travel recommendations for the disabled

1 — Anticipate and prepare for medical problems

2 — Consider a medical check-up before departure

3 — Warn airline of special medical, dietary or mobility requirements. Complete MEDIF for air travel

4 — Organise vaccination and prophylaxis

5 — Pre-book aircraft seating

6 — Continue routine medication en route and carry it in hand luggage

7 — Purchase adequate, inclusive medical insurance

8 — Exercise the legs whenever possible in flight

9 — Drink plenty of water and juices on board

10— Avoid pulses, salads and alcohol with in-flight meals

11— Rest up after arrival at destination if journey crosses many time zones

12— Consider availability of rampage; lifts, wheelchair lifts, lavatory access, size and supports; wheelchair availability on board; facilities at transit airports

Coach travel

Pre-enquiry must encompass availability of a mechanical wheelchair lift, consider employees willingness to manually lift patients on board and adequate access for the wheelchair to onboard toilet.

Sea travel

It was once the policy of almost all cruise liners to discourage the disabled traveller from taking a cruise for reasons of safety, insurance and legal liability, but new ships have been refurbished with the disabled person in mind.

Ships devoid of lifts can prove an insurmountable hazard for those with fixed knees and hip deformities. Stairs and companionways can be narrow and steep on board ship and six or seven deck levels are commonplace. Transit of these areas in a swaying vessel is likely to promote falls in the unstable. The use of a wheelchair is perhaps a wise precaution to ensure extra stability fo those with loss of mobility or balance problems.

Wheelchair users will be expected to be accompanied by a companion responsible for any assistance needed. Sleeping accommodation should ensure wheelchair access to toilets, proximity to elevators, access to the decks and provision of a bath rather than a shower.

Train transportation

Train transportation must include easy access from platform to carriage with available porterage. In Britain, even on mainline trains, half the wheelchair travellers often have to make the journey in the guard's van. In the absence of a guard, the only lifeline may be a tenuous telephone link with the driver. Toilet access may also prove impossible, either being too small or not accessible. Travel health consultants should advise the disabled that journeys be planned for off-peak periods when staff are less likely to be overworked. However, in a study of disabled rail travellers who had actually informed British Rail that they were travelling, one third found they received insufficient assistance on the journey (Automobile Association 1992). About half of the sample who used buses and trains in the UK admitted to difficulties in getting on and off the vehicle. Advantage should be taken of pre-boarding to avoid congestion and the special booklets provided by the Air Transport Users Committee and by airports.

Speedy transit will determine most incapacitated patients will use airline travel. Maintaining continence looms large in the mind of many handicapped travellers but careful pre-planning will allow full use of the available facilities. However, many public toilets are devoid of wall supports or grab rails and in may parts of the world the sanitary ware may be of the 'hole in the ground' variety, quite unsuited for use by the disabled. These inadequacies may be insurmountable obstacles for the disabled traveller but for the majority with frailties, pre-planning and organisation will invariably smooth the way to a safer journey.

Table 9.4: Management of the disabled potential traveller

1 — Clinically examine high risk patients

2 — Review routine drug therapy

3 — Advise need for special adjustments eg. to diet, to inflight therapy, eg. insulin

4 — Stress need to carry and maintain medication en route

5 — Organise appropriate vaccinations and prophylaxis

6 — Advise patient to report invalid status to the airline, shipping or railway agents

7 — Counsel on special risks of altitude, extremes of heat and cold, immobility, cabin air pressure and humidity, jet-lag and effects of environmental disturbance

8 — Stress need for adequate inclusive holiday medical insurance cover

9 — Discuss availability of medical facilities and disabled aids at airports, train and coach stations, transit stopovers

10— Points for consideration with air travel

- is the individual fit to fly;
- will passenger be acceptable to the airline;
- has the patient completed IATAS MEDIF information form
- What physical defects are there
  - i) in sight
  - ii) hearing
  - iii) mental faculty
  - iv) limb deformities
- fixed joints
- spasticity;
- is the patient going to be accompanied;
- is the patient continent

World travel is feasible for the disabled on individualised journeys. They must be guided by health counsellors towards realistic goals and are well advised to travel with a spouse or independent supporter. They may require special medical counselling and guidance towards support organisations for further advice. Safe travel for the handicapped passenger demands careful pre-travel planning, competent medical assessment, sound counselling and a realistic venue. Within these parameters, world travel need not elude the determined incapacitated traveller.

Useful addresses:

RADAR (Royal Association for the Disabled and Rehabilitation) 25, Mortimer Street, London W1N 8AD
Moore, U S A - Mobility International U S A, P O Box 3511, Eugene, Oregon 97403

References

Automobile Assoc^{n} (1992). Mobility for All: Disabled Travellers and their needs, AA Basingstoke.
British Airways - *Blind flying*, tape cassette, in association with the Royal Society for the Blind
Dawood, R (3rd edn). *How to stay healthy abroad*, 445-450, Oxford University Press
Green L (1977). Carriage of invalid passengers by air, *Br J Hosp Med, 32-37*
McIntosh I (1988). Care of the disabled traveller, *Scot Med*, Dec, 9-11
McIntosh I (1992). *Travel and health in the elderly: A medical handbook*, Quay Publishing, Lancaster
Stone D (1991). Keeping a lookout for visual impairment, *Med Monitor*, 47

CHAPTER 10

HEALTH HAZARDS AND WATER SPORTS ABROAD

Summary

Water sports provide a great attraction for many who holiday abroad. Warm seas, shelving beaches, roaring surf, trade winds, racing rivers and winding waterways each attract the enthusiast. Expert and novice, intent on sailing, surfing, canoeing, rafting, windsurfing and water-skiing throng the shore line and dot the seas. Less intrepid holiday-makers, overheated by tropical and Mediterranean sun, plunge into swimming and rock pools, lochs, lakes and lagoons to sport themselves and cool off. On, in and beneath the water, tourists thrust through, over and under the waves. Many do so unaware of the health hazards associated with water sports and the particular dangers to which they expose themselves in foreign places and exotic climes.

Each year there are avoidable deaths from trauma and disease. Drowning, hypothermia, diving injuries, boating and surfing accidents take a remorseless toll of travellers' lives. Sports-induced infections can cause acute and chronic disease and prolonged morbidity. An awareness of risk and simple precautions can save life or prevent spoiled holidays.

Swimming pools

For swimmers, water in a river, lake or open sea demands respect as a potent source of hazard. Even neglected foreign swimming pools have to be treated with caution. The safest swimming place is a chlorinated hotel pool but if inadequately treated with chemicals, it may be polluted or harbour bilharzia.

Tragically, young people break their necks and are killed or paralysed regularly by diving too steeply into unsuspectedly shallow pools (Grundy *et al*, 1991). The majority are men with an average age of 24 years and many have been drinking alcohol before they dive. A recent Scottish survey recorded that the most common location for this kind of injury was Spain and Greece. The bone injury is usually a crush fracture of a lower cervical vertebra, usually C5, with direct injury to the cord. Fatality and tetraplegia might be avoided if swimmers shunned alcohol before taking to the water, looking before they dive, refraining from diving into less than 1.5m of water and using a flat projectory dive.

Freshwater swimming, away from the hotel has its own inherent dangers. Many popular world-wide coastal resorts now have sewage-polluted coastal waters and conjunctivitis and ear infections can result. Swimmers in the Mediterranean have been shown to have more gastrointestinal upsets than non-swimmers. Algal bloom (Dunlop, 1991) can frequently contaminate freshwater lakes as well as maritime waters. The blue-green algae (cyano bacteria) can be toxic and swimmers should avoid contact with algal scum and the water around it. Exposure to water contaminated with rat urine may also expose the swimmer or water sportsman to leptospirosis (Wolkans *et al*, 1988).

Case History 10.1

Two British travellers set off independently to travel the world and met on a wooden raft expedition in Thailand. The raft capsized and they swallowed a considerable amount of river water. A week later both were admitted to a Bangkok hospital with the abrupt onset of severe headache, myalgia and high fever. No diagnosis was made and they were discharged after a few days and returned to Britain. Within days of each other they were admitted independently to an infectious disease unit of an English hospital with aseptic meningitis as a result of leptospirosis.

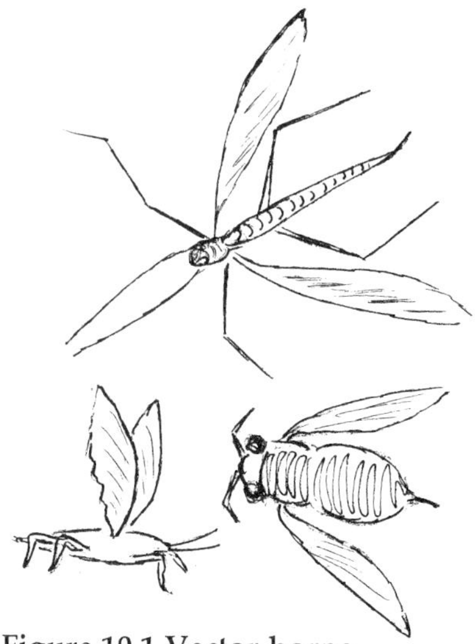

Figure 10.1 Vector-borne Diseases

Monsoon rains can flush out bank rodents and their nests, and heavily contaminate river water with leptospires. Through much of Africa and the Middle East, lakes and pools are infected with bilharzia (schistosomiasis). The eggs of the intestinal worms hatch in water and infect certain kinds of snails. The larvae develop in the host and multiply with some swimming free to seek out and penetrate the skin of a human host. In much of Africa, parts of the Middle East and Brazil, the majority of the population is infected. All those who swim in infected streams, rivers and lakes or indulge in water sports, especially where there are large areas of surface water, are at risk of infection. Even deep water, far off-shore is not safe. Lagoons can harbour S mansoni and even small patches of water far divorced from human habitation can be infected. It should never be assumed that fresh water is free from infection in an endemic area. Salt water, brackish water and chlorinated water are safe but neglected swimming pools can become colonised by the snails. Rubber boots and wet suits offer protection for the water sportsman but external clothing must be dried quickly in the sun immediately after use. Artificial man-made lakes are particularly notorious for the risk of infection.

Dangerous fish

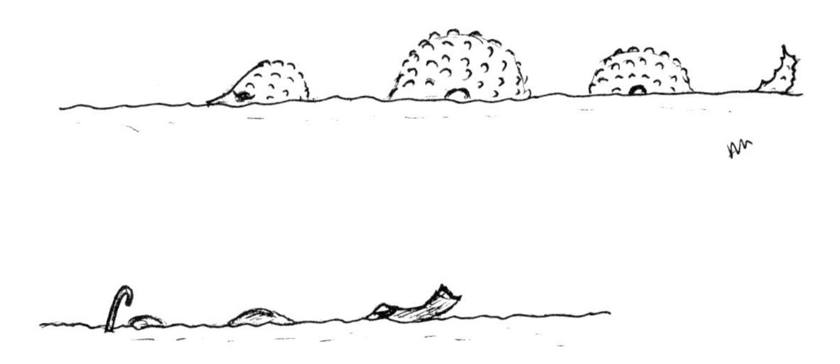

Figure 10.2 Hazards of Watersports

'Swimmers itch' is caused by schistosome larvae which have penetrated the skin and died there. They do not develop further and cause an intense itch, a variety of cercarial dermatitis. It can occur in temperate as well as tropical countries and also in the USA. Fortunately, antihistamine tablets or ointment is all that is required for treatment. Unknown foreign waters do not only bring the risk of attack by sharks, groupers, stingrays and crocodiles, they also present off-shore winds, underground swells, thundering surf and treacherous currents, all additional risks for the unwary swimmer. There is the ever-present risk of drowning and hypothermia can strike in colder waters. Menstruating women may be apprehensive that menstrual blood may attract predators but sharks and piranha are not attracted when blood is absorbed into sanitary towels or tampons. In parts of Southeast Asia where they are prevalent, aquatic leeches will gorge on any unprotected flesh. They will crawl into the mouth, nostrils and eyes and are best avoided by refraining from swimming in forest pools and streams. Many fish and also sea anemones can inflict painful and dangerous stings. The coelenterates possess stings, especially on the tentacles. Contact results in severe burning pain followed by erythema and weals. With extensive stings from the Portuguese man of war, collapse may follow. Abrasions from corals can cause ulcers which can take weeks to heal.

Diving hazards

Brilliantly hued fish beneath the waves, entice the swimmer and tempt many into snorkelling, an apparently benign underwater pursuit. Use of a goggle without a nose piece, however, risks blood-shot or black eyes. Hyperventilation in an effort to prolong the dive before starting is hazardous for it delays the build up of carbon dioxide. The snorkeller may use up all his oxygen and lose consciousness before the urge to surface and breathe again is felt. Hyperventilation before a dive has led to many deaths from drowning.

Sub aqua

Sub aqua enthusiasts are attracted to the Caribbean and Red Sea where warm, clear waters can tempt even experienced divers into the indiscretion of deeper dives and nitrogen narcosis (Demberg, 1987). This is a physiological phenomenon of aqualung diving, not an irreversible pathological condition. When diving deeper than 16m with compressed air the high absolute partial pressures of nitrogen in the compressed air cause light-headedness, giddiness and impairment of concentration which disappear on returning to the surface. However, an intoxicated diver can act in a bizarre way when experiencing the 'Rapture of the Deep', disregarding safe diving principles and ignoring safe ascent procedures, thus incurring decompression sickness (Stewart, 1989). This is caused by the formation and circulation of bubbles of nitrogen gas which come out of solution and the body tissues during ascent. The bubbles form if the diver is submerged for a relatively long time or ascends too fast to allow for the nitrogen dissolved in the tissues to remain in solution in the blood stream and eventually be exhaled. They can occlude small arteries and veins and cause physiological dysfunction in joints and bones, the central nervous system and the lungs. Divers visiting developing countries may find equipment less than reliable and compressed air supplies of variable quality. Novice divers can be encouraged to undertake dives without adequate training and supervision, and gastrointestinal upset, the scourge of the traveller, can be dangerous if individuals dive when affected. Abdominal cramps, dehydration and diarrhoea and fever, which are not uncommon in foreign travel, are contraindications to safe diving.

Hypothermia

Even in tropical waters, hypothermia can develop if only a light shirt and trunks are worn. If water temperature is less than 21°C protective suits must be worn. An unclad swimmer in water at a lower temperature than this will lose heat faster than the body can create it, as water conducts heat 25 times more rapidly than air. Chilling and hypothermia can soon follow. It is known that an unprotected swimmer at 5°C will be endangered within 20 minutes of entering the water and will be dead within one hour and forty minutes. Temperature drops with increasing depth, the greatest change occurring after the first 10m descent below which the sun's warming effects cease to operate.

Scuba-divers risk decompression sickness if they fly home immediately after a dive. Aircraft cabin pressure will allow enough of a pressure gradient between lesser cabin ambient pressure and higher tissue pressures of nitrogen remaining from the dive, to cause some bubble formation and subsequent decompression sickness. No dive greater than 9m should be taken within 24 hours of a flight and, even after shallow no-decompression dives, at least 12 hours should lapse before flying.

Pulmonary problems

Easy access to scuba facilities attracts novices to the sport. Standards of equipment and instruction on diving safety are often much below those of the UK. Novice divers in foreign resorts may be taught by ill-qualified instructors and language constraints may cause communications difficulties. A quick financial return is often sought by diving operators and instruction may comprise a short, superficial programme designed only to get the novice to pay the fee, get into the gear and plunge into the water. Inadequate instruction at the very earliest stage can be hazardous and the diver may risk barotrauma even when practising in deeper swimming pools. If novice aqualung divers hold their breath during a rapid ascent from depth, air embolism, pneumothorax and mediastinal emphysema can result. Expanding air inside the lungs may rupture the alveoli with tracking of the air into the pulmonary venous system and interstitial tissues. Warm foreign waters entice women to explore under the water and women divers with significant pre-menstrual symptoms should not dive as severe cramps can effect concentration and mimic signs of decompression sickness (McIntosh, 1991). Pregnant women are advised not to dive at all as little is known of the potential dangerous effects on the developing fetus.

Asthmatic divers are at special risk as many are unaware that they should not dive for 48 hours after a wheezy attack (Farrell and Glanville, 1990). Optimum diving conditions abroad will encourage the wheezy diver into following his sport when mildly wheezy. There is a risk of sections of lung being incompletely ventilated as the diver ascends and the sections may fail to empty sufficiently resulting in pneumothorax or even gas embolism (Douglas, 1983).

Divers using borrowed equipment can now be reassured regarding the risk of AIDS infection. The UK Health and Safety Executive has just published 'AIDS, HIV Infection and Diving' which confirms that HIV cannot be transmitted by breathing apparatus or during the first-aid procedures taught to divers.

Surfing and sail-board problems

The sight of experienced surfers, 'hotdogging' across the face of a 10-foot curl on a breaking wave attracts many to this sport. Injuries are common, especially in the novice, usually as a result of being struck by his own or someone else's board. Abrasions and gravel burns are common. Body surfers are, however, at greatest risk of severe injury (Harris, 1980). Injuries are sustained when the wave is steep and breaks precipitously; the resulting wave is known as a 'dumper' and injury results from the individual being rammed head first onto the seabed like a pile driver. The neck is forcefully flexed and rotated and fractures of the skull and cervical spine are common. Steep dives at the water's edge can also force the head on to an unsuspected sandbank with resultant fracture and the likelihood of tetraplegia.

Windsurfing is a popular pastime but collapsing booms, falling masts and frequent capsize make the sport potentially hazardous. Even in the tropics sailors clad only

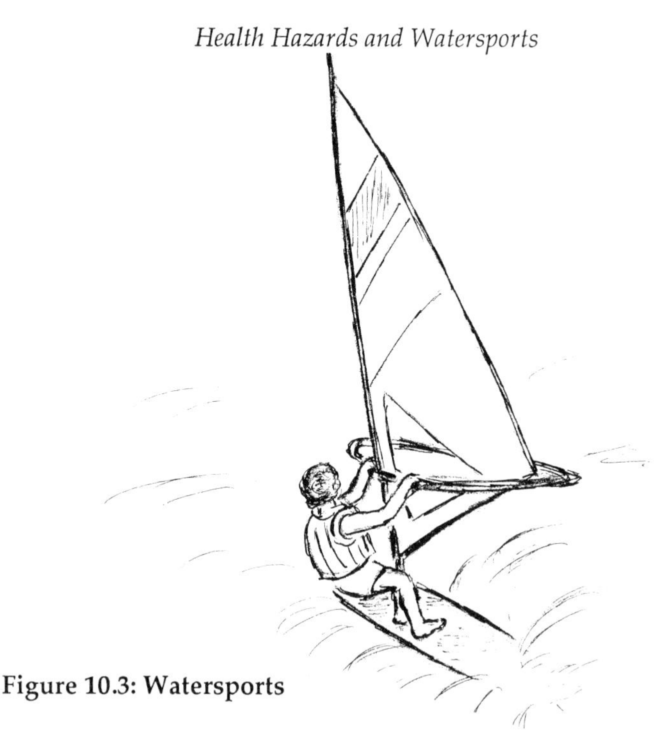

Figure 10.3: Watersports

in swimsuits can suffer from hypothermia and fatigue. Exhaustion can overcome them if the board is swept out to sea. Novice windsurfers should always sail into the wind and along the shores. Falls off surf boards into shallow lagoons may also impale the feet on sea urchins' spines which can penetrate even plastic beach shoes.

Water-skiing

Water-skiing attracts the young traveller. Off crowded holidays beaches, collision with other skiers and swimmers is always a possibility. Skiers also risk contact with algal waters and with algal bloom which can be present in fresh, esturine and marine waters, and can result in pneumonia. Women water-skiers risk foreign-body penetration of the vagina and high-speed vaginal douching in falls from the skis. The inrush of contaminated water can promote

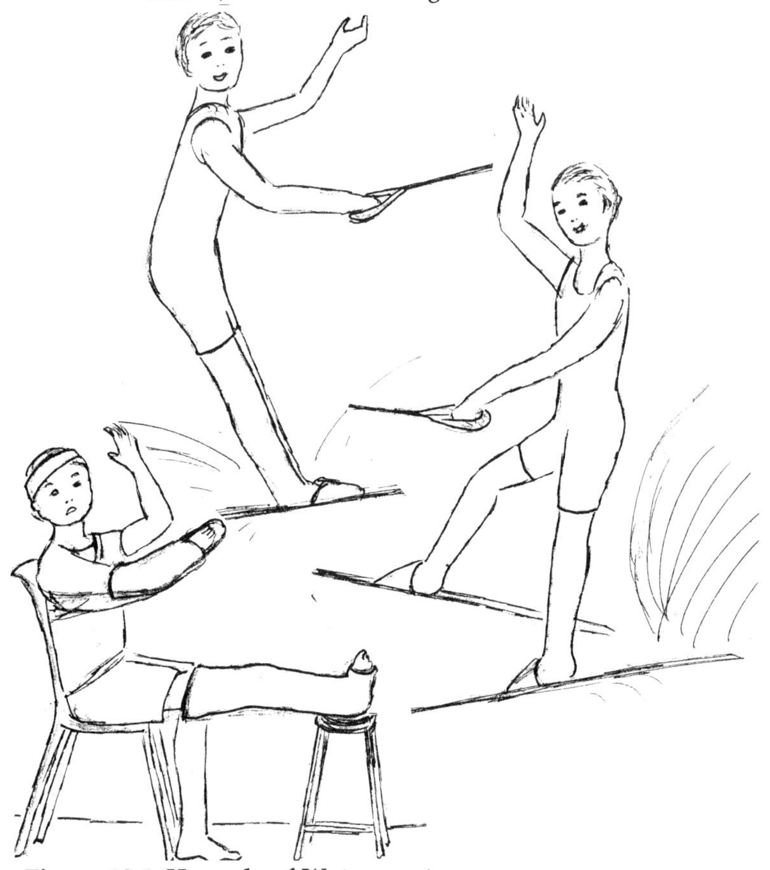

Figure 10.4: Hazards of Watersports

ascending infections and they should wear adequate costumes covering the perineum.

Barefoot water-skiing has its devotees and it requires much skill and courage as the tow boat has to be travelling at a minumum speed of 45mph. The sport has its share of spinal cord injuries. The perineum can be traumatised by water hitting it at high speed. Sudden catastrophic failure of wet-suit stitching results in high-speed rectal and vaginal douching; rectal and vaginal tears and salpingitis are recorded.

Case history 10.2

An orthopaedic surgeon has graphically recorded the massive muscle breakdown and bruising from the high speed barrage of water which he experienced, while endeavouring to learn the art of barefoot skiing. He developed haematuria and myoglobinuria as a result. Adequate body protection must be worn in this sport and is easily forgotten in the warm waters of a tropical resort (Barrat, 1990).

Small boat risks

Small boats have their enthusiasts and they throng holiday beaches. Canoeists are recorded as having developed pneumonia from algal-covered waters and there are reports of leptospirosis in those canoeing in rat-infested waters. The organisms of Leptrospira interrogans complex can enter the body through a cut or an abrasion, or more commonly, through the gastrointestinal tract. Small sailboats, pedalos, rowing boats and yachts are hired out at every holiday resort. Swinging booms knock sailors into the water and render them unconscious, and fast currents or tidal races sweep them away. The risk of drowning, exposure and dehydration are constant reminders that water sports demand caution and safety awareness.

Risks for on-shore water enthusiasts

On-shore water-side enthusiasts risk infection from larva migrans. The hookworm larva infects the sand above the waterline. Discarded from the intestine of dogs and cats, it burrows into human skin and, although it cannot develop further, it wanders under the skin causing red itchy lines (Verbov, 1989). Infection can be avoided by wearing sandals on the beach. However, all who expose themselves by sea or in the sea, risk contact with mosquitoes and sand-flies and other airborne vectors. Exposure of large areas of skin by those indulging in water sports brings the risk of serious sunburn and many forget that the rays penetrate through water and thin blouses and shirts.

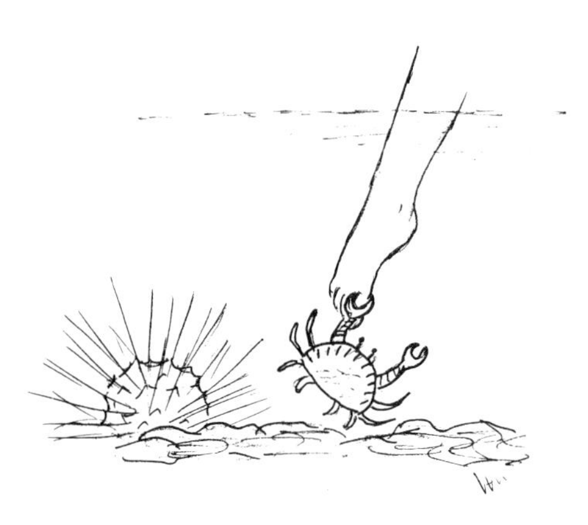

Sea-side Hazards

Table 10.1: Water sports health hazards

Drowning	
Hypothermia	
Skeletal injury	spinal fractures sports trauma
Infections	cyano bacterial infection leptospirosis bilharzia gastroenteritis casualty treatment risks HIV infection hepatitis
Tissue damage	fish bite larva migrans infestation leech bites jelly fish stings coral abrasions gravel burns sea urchin spine penetration
Decompression sickness	
Hyperventilation anoxia	
Foreign body penetration of vagina	
Pelvic inflammatory disease	
Sun burn	

Management

Identify the sport
Advise on health hazards
Suggest the traveller carries an anti HIV first aid kit
Encourage the use of very high factor sunblocks
Ensure tetanus vaccination protection
Suggest the wearing of canvas shoes on beaches and for swimming

Despite this catalogue of morbid possibilities, the majority of tourists travel the world and enjoy water sports, relatively free from major health disturbance. An awareness of potential hazard and maintenance of sensible safety precautions, with a constant appreciation of risk and respect for strange waters, will allow most to enjoy the waters of the world in safety. It behoves the travel health counsellor to identify potential hazards. With forewarning, many sporting mishaps might be avoided.

References

Barrat D S (1990). Can orthopaedic surgeons walk on water? *Br Med J*, **301**, 1429-30.
Demberg M L (1987). Health advice for the travelling scuba-diver, *Trav Med Intl*, **6:2**, 61-65.
Douglas D M (1983). Shallow water air diving, *Scot Med*, **August** 18-19.
Dunlop J (1991). Blooming alga, *Br Med J*, **302**, 671-672
Farrell S and Glanville P (1990). Diving practices of scuba divers with asthma, *Br Med J*, **300,** 166.
Grundy D, Penny P and Graham L (1991). Diving into the unknown, *Br Med J*, **302**, 670-671.
Harries M G (1980). Surfing and surfing injuries, *Medisport*, **2:4**, 106-107.
Health and Safety Executive 1991). Ref. IND (G)101L 11991, United Kingdom.
McIntosh I B (1991). The health of the woman traveller, *Trav Med Intl*, **9:1**, 24-28.
Stewart K (1989). The rapture of the deep, *Scot Med*, August, 8-10.
Verbov J (1989). Skin hazards of travel, *Trav Med Intl*, **7:4**, 143-147.
Wolkans E, Cope A and Waitkins S (1988). Rapids, rafts and rats, *The Lancet*, 283-284.

CHAPTER 11

HIGH ALTITUDE, HIGH RISK TRAVEL

Summary

Ease of travel, improved access and the quest for adventure result in ever more people travelling to the world's highest altitudes. They risk acute mountain sickness and cardiac and pulmonary stress. With sound advice, timely acclimatisation and appropriate prophylaxis those who wish to venture high can do so in relative safety.

The number of tourists, trekkers and mountaineers exposing themselves to high altitude in the Himalayas and Andes is increasing. Thousands of trekkers and hundreds of climbers now climb to the limits of human habitation and many venture far beyond to the summits of the world's highest mountains. Many of these adventurers have a limited awareness of the dangers of hypoxia associated with high climbing. Doctors attached to mountaineering groups are usually aware of the fatal potential of acute mountain illness.

High altitude effects

General practitioners are less likely to be cognisant with the dangers of high altitude exposure. Trekking groups to the world's high mountains, constrained by time, continue to press on regardless, maintaining upward progress to the advantage of the whole group and the dangerous detriment of individuals affected by acute mountain sickness (AMS).

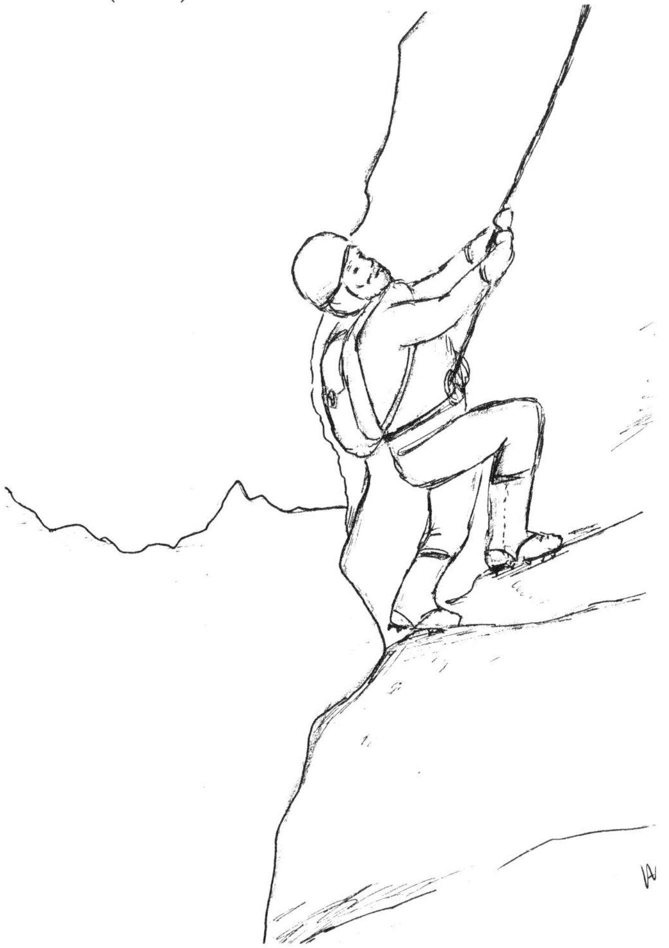

Figure 11.1: High Altitude Illness

Case history 11.1

Recently, the expedition doctor of a large commercially organised tourist group in Bhutan allowed trekkers with worsening symptoms of AMS to continue over increasingly higher passes. The year previously, a group had to be air-lifted out of the same area after a long delay, when snow and storm had cut them off. If these unwell trekkers had developed severe and death threatening AMS, rapid descent might have been impracticable, timely air rescue unlikely and preventable deaths a strong possibility. An inexperienced leader and novice mountaineering doctor took unjustifiable risks to keep the party intact and advancing on schedule.

Risks of AMS

In one reported survey in Nepal, the overall incidence of AMS was 53 percent and, although only 4.3 percent had life-threatening illness, these incidents resulted in dangerous, difficult and expensive rescues which might have been avoided. If due attention and treatment had been provided for those with early symptoms, the severe manifestations of more acute and potentially fatal illness might have been prevented.

A university research evaluation of seven cases of fatal AMS concluded that more medical advice should be given to those embarking on strenuous and sporting high altitude holidays. Trek companies tend to minimise risks to prospective clients and the burden of explanation falls upon family physicians. However, limitations of knowledge regarding predictive indicators, pre-emptive diagnosis and treatment can dilute the benefits of such attempts at education; a fact brought home by the revelation that in the investigated group, three of those who died were doctors.

Packaged treks and tours, speedy air travel, transit to airfields situated above 3,000 metres and improved access to global high places ensure that many more people will suffer from the minor and major effects of altitude with every passing year. Eager trekkers and climbers expose themselves to the rigours of the heights and a condition which is poorly understood, despite intensive study.

Not only are young trekkers and ardent mountaineers exposed to AMS, conventional tourists can be affected. Flights into Mexico City and many South American airports in the Andes may land at airports at high altitude. Tourists visiting Inca settlements like Machu Piccu in Peru, or Lake Titicaca in Bolivia find themselves gasping for air when leaving the aircraft. They can be badly affected by the effects of the low partial pressure of oxygen experienced at high altitude if undertaking undue exercise or up-hill walking. Several regular, scheduled bus and train services traverse passes high enough to promote anoxia in normally healthy European travellers. The cardio-pulmonary compromised, the pregnant and the elderly traveller can be placed at marked health risk while often unaware of the hazard to health the journey entails. On several South American railway trains, cylinder oxygen is routinely offered to passengers crossing the highest routes. The Everest tourist hotel, on the walking route into the world's highest mountain, recognised the dangers to its clients of thin air and installed piped oxygen into bedrooms catering for the anoxic.

Case history 12.2

An elderly female patient intent on following in the footsteps of the Incas, flew to Cusco in Peru, a former city of the Inca empire. At 3,800 metres altitude she became breathless, dizzy, developed chest pain and collapsed in the foyer of the hotel while booking in. She spent her time in the city, curtailed to bed-rest and breathing intermittent oxygen as a supplement at night. Her long-anticipated journey of a life-time almost ended in disaster. Neither the GP who had provided her vaccinations or her travel agent had warned her of potential risks of higher altitude exposure.

History

The effect of high altitude on man has been recognised for centuries. In 326 BC, Alexander the Great recorded the untoward effect of high altitude on his troops when crossing the Hindu Kush into India. He blamed it upon the unsteadiness of the atmosphere and the ancient Chinese referred to the Himalayas as the Greater and Lesser Headache Peaks. The first clinical description of AMS was given by a Jesuit priest, Father D'Acosta, in the 16th century when he crossed the Andes. The first comprehensive account of the malady was given by Sir Joseph Barcroft in 1921-22 who described the illness in passengers travelling from the Pacific coast into the Andes by train to a height of 3,000m in a few hours. More recently, in 1962, the Indian army discovered it had lost more soldiers from acute mountain sickness than to battle wounds in the war against the Chinese .

For a long time, it was believed that the condition resulted from exposure to rock-bearing ores of antimony and lead which gave the condition its alternative name of Soroche. The true pathophysiology still remains unknown although hypoxia appears to be the symptom trigger in association with large shifts of fluid from extracellular to intracellular spaces.

There is as yet, no absolute predictive measure to identify those likely to suffer from exposure to high altitude. In recent years it has been recognised that there is a spectrum of high altitude disease, resulting from hypoxia, with symptoms ranging from the trivial and self-limiting to the serious and life-threatening. There can be remarkably little difference in initial presentation.

Physiology

By general acceptance, high altitude is defined as heights over 3,000m and it is over this level that symptoms of AMS appear. Normal partial pressure of oxygen at sea-level is 140mmHg and this drops proportionately with elevation, so that at 3,500m individuals are exposed to a pressure of 103mm, a mere 65 percent of that at sea-level. At this altitude there is a physiological response of hyperventilation accompanied by respiratory alkalosis and pulmonary hypertension, with an increase in cardiac rate, a 25 percent fall in stroke volume and a similar percentage rise in cerebral blood flow. A stay at this level will bring fluid retention and increased red cell production with polycythaemia.

Acclimatisation

Acclimatisation is the physiological response to the stress of altitude. Slow acclimatisation with its resultant increase in blood oxygen-carrying capacity decreases the risk of succumbing to AMS in most people. However, 'Alpine-push' techniques are currently used on many mountain assaults. Commercially-packaged, high 'fly-ins' are enthusiastically embraced by time-constrained back-packers. This speedier mountain access makes it less likely that those at risk take advantage of this physiological response. Many now ignore traditional rest days and acclimatisation halts with relative impunity but the substantial number who begin high mountain trips unacclimatised to hypobaric hypoxia do so at their peril.

A study of trekkers in 1986 (Kayser) crossing the Thorung Pass (5,400), the highest point on the popular Annapurna Ciruit in Nepal, found that nearly two thirds were suffering from AMS. Pollard has noted that it is common on this trail to meet trekkers with AMS. Too ill to walk, they are carried by porters over high passes so as not to inconvenience other walkers in the group by forcing a return to base.

Signs and symptoms of AMS

At the minor end of the spectrum, AMS is now considered a self-limiting form of cerebral oedema with hypoxia playing the primary part but exacerbated by strenuous exercise. The symptoms are malaise, nausea, headache and breathlessness which present within 36 hours of arrival at altitude. This symptomology is at best an inconvenience, always unpleasant and sometimes very debilitating. Providing the afflicted rest and do not climb higher, the effects disappear in a few days; there is little risk of fatal sequelae and the person can then climb higher.

Table 11.1: Signs and symptoms

— headache
— nausea
— anorexia
— dizziness
— dyspnoea
— insomnia

HAPO

It is now recognised that high altitude pulmonary oedema (HAPO) is an extension of AMS, often presenting within the same time scale. The patient develops breathlessness at rest, rapidly becomes severely short of breath and cyanosed, and has a frothy, blood-stained sputum. The course of the illness can proceed apace and soon be fatal.

HACO

A serious concomitant presentation of AMS is high altitude cerebral oedema (HACO) which can coexist with HAPO. Headache is constant, severe and unrelieved by analgesia, and there is usually ataxia, crippling lassitude and symptoms normally associated at sea level with raised intracranial pressure. The patient can deteriorate very rapidly into stupor, coma and death within hours.

Initially these manifestations of potentially fatal illness are so similar to benign AMS that the high risk patient is not always identified or pulmonary symptoms are taken for pneumonia and mistreated. Ataxia and early papilloedema are cardinal signs of fatal illness and, when elicited, descent of the invalid to lower altitude is mandatory.

Table 11.2: People at high risk from high altitude exposure

- Those who have previously experienced AMS
- Those with myocardial insufficiency
- The anaemic
- Individuals suffering from chronic obstructive airways disease
- Those with cerebro-vascular insufficiency
- Sufferers from stroke disease
- Pregnant women
- Patients on respiratory depressant drugs

Treatment

AMS responds rapidly with descent which is not, however, always practicable in high-mountain climes and terrain. Oxygen by face-mask should be given when available. Double-blind studies have shown the benefit of dexamethasone administration in severe cases. Acetazolamide alleviates some symptoms, especially the headache, but diuretics are of no proven value. Exposure to higher partial pressures of oxygen as soon as possible is the prerequisite to cure.

Many first-time altitude exlorers approach family and expedition doctors asking if they will be fit to climb high and if they can avoid AMS. There are no absolute predictive factors to guide the response. Physical fitness does not preclude onset of AMS. Younger age groups seem to be at higher risk but this may simply be that they travel too fast, too high and too quickly. A good diuresis experienced on ascent is considered a sign of acclimatisation but its absence is a poor indicator of susceptibility. Previous trouble-free high altitude exposure suggests problem-free re-exposure to the same altitude but there is no guarantee of this.

In cardiac terms, the mass of accumulated data does not suggest that high altitude alone threatens the normal heart, inducing it to fail or infarct. There are several recorded instances of patients who have recovered from coronary bypass surgery and then climbed safely to 5750m in Nepal, but our current state of knowledge allows no accurate predictions about the risks taken by someone with heart disease exposed to these heights. It would be wise to warn off those with angina and myocardial ischaemia although hypertension is not a contraindication to high altitude travel. Little is known about drug metabolism in hypoxic states but drugs with respiratory depressant effects should not be taken in the mountains. Women should stop oral contraceptive ingestion before venturing to a great height.

Acetazolamide prophylaxis

Acetazolamide is now favoured by tour groups and back-packers as a useful prophylactic to prevent the onset of AMS. Placebo and controlled within-group studies on Kilimanjaro lend support to its efficacy in preventing and alleviating symptoms at the minor end of the AMS spectrum (Green 1981; McIntosh 1986). There is no conclusive evidence that it prevents progression to fatal forms of the disease. The drug is a carbonic anhydrase inhibitor with a mild diuretic action and its effective function in AMS is probably the result of increased tissue oxygenation. It should be taken 24 hours before exposure to altitudes above 3,500m and, except for a tingling paraesthesia of fingers and feet, appears to have no adverse side-effects.

Table 11.3: Management of high altitude travellers

- — Advise on dangers
- — discourage high risk people from going too high
- — offer prophylaxis to those staying above 2500m
- — advise on staged, slow upwards ascent
- — advise need for descent if worsening symptoms
- — **Rate of ascent:** Ideally, for trekking above 3,000m, ascent should be at the rate of 300m per day for 2 days, followed by 150m per day (Milledge 1983). This is an unconstrained progress and much depends upon the terrain to be covered, which will often prove to be a series of ascents and descents on the usual mountain approach. The main consideration is for the climber not to go too fast, too high and too far each day. Acclimatisation usually takes about three weeks.
- — Check for anaemia
- — Check for history of angina, bronchospasm, obstructive airways disease, myocardial and cerebrovascular insufficiency
- — Exclude pregnancy
- — Clinical examination if cardio-pulmonary problems in the past
- — Offer prophylaxis

Case history 12.3

One of my patients developed severe headache, nausea, vomiting and breathlessness when driven by car without stopping, on a day traverse from Marrakesh to the oasis of Oarzazate in the Sahara. The high passes of the Atlas Mountains climb above 2,500 metres and her symptoms occurred each time she ventured to cross the watershed. But for a slight headache, the symptoms did not appear when she took acetazoleamide as prophylaxis. She developed identical symptoms, however, some years later when crossing the American Rockies in a bus without prophylaxis.

Conclusion

High altitude climbing is now big business, vital to the tourist industry of many developing countries, and package tours are possible to nine of the world's highest mountains. Once aboard the jet liner, those who wish can be climbing within 24 hours in the higher Himalayas at a potentially dangerous altitude. Ease of travel, improved access, financial affluence and the quest for adventure will result in more people travelling to the highest altitudes and risking AMS and cardiac stress. Sound advice, leisurely ascent, timely acclimatisation and appropriate drug prophylaxis can ensure that those who venture high can do so in relative safety.

References

Bacharach A L and Edholm O G (1965). *Exploration Medicine,* Wright and Sons, Bristol

D'Costa J (1880). History of the Andes, Haklyut Society

Ellis F, Ellis M *et al* (1988). Stress factors and AMS, *Trav Med Intl,* **6**, 99-104

Green M, Kerr A and McIntosh I (1981). Acetazolamide in AMS, A double-blind study, *Br Med J,* **283**, 811-113

Kayser B (1991). AMS in Western Tourists with the Thorung Pass, *J Wilderness Med,* **2**, 110-117

McIntosh I and Prescott R (1986). Acetazolamide in prevention of AMS, *J Intl Med Res,* **14**, 285-287

Milledge J (1983). Acute Mountain Sickness, *Thorax,* **38**, 641

Oelz O (1988). Treatment of AMS with dexamethasone, *Trav Med Intl,* **6**, 94

Rennie D (1989). Will mountaineers have heart attacks: *J Amer Med Assoc,* **261**, 1045-6

Ward M P (1975). *Mountain Medicine,* Crossby Lockwood Stables, St Albans

CHAPTER 12

EXPEDITION MEDICINE

Summary

Expedition treks and tours may offer subsidised travel to alluring far-away places for the impecunious doctor with a yearn for adventure, but those tempted should beware. Careful choice of travel group is vital if one is to avoid medical mishaps and ensure an optimum of leisure and pleasure on such a working holiday.

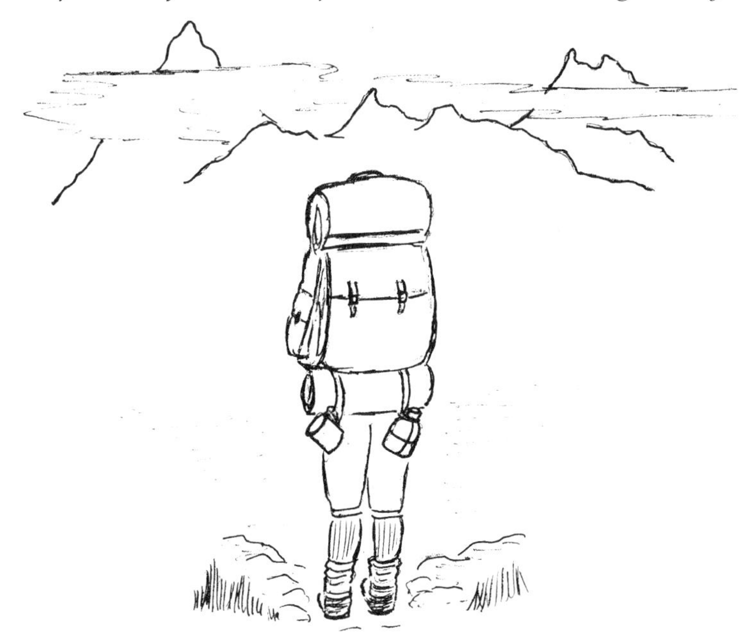

Figure 12.1: The Backpack Expeditioner

Introduction

This topic embraces elements of medicine which create problems on expeditions to the world's remote and/or high places. Trauma infection, hypo and hyperthermia, altitude sickness and insect bites have all to be considered. Travel sickness and the risk from road traffic accident loom large in expeditions over rough or mountainous roads. Back packers run a higher risk of succumbing to hepatitis and in the young, the AIDS risk may be relevant.

Far from hospital or medical facilities, the burden of care falls on the expedition medical officer who often is dependent upon the medication and equipment that he or she alone can carry into the wilderness. Small is beautiful when it comes to the expedition first aid kit, but appropriate contents are crucial to successful medical management on the trail.

Solo expeditioners and adventurers often approach GPs for information on special vaccinations, prophylaxis and health advice. Their trips may be through jungles, deserts, the tropics, high mountains and as far afield as the Arctic and Antarctica. Their wanderings will present potentially high hazards to health.

Enterprising groups entice doctors to join expeditions and commit themselves to the party's medical care. Often an undemanding task, the responsibilities can prove onerous. Divorced or distanced from conventional medical facilities with professional support days away, the expedition medical officer has to be prepared for every eventuality. He or she may need to be a resourceful surgeon, physician, psychiatrist and even an obstetrician.

My own expedition experiences often stretched my medical expertise to the limit and called for ingenuity and skills rarely required in general medical practice. The following anecdotes and management tips may prepare the novice expedition medic for the rigours often met en route. However, no matter how well prepared the expedition for medical emergency, the novel and the unexpected are sure to befall the accompanying doctor. On a recent trip to Zimbabwe when the main medical hazard appeared to come from the rocks and crocodiles met in rafting down the rapids of the Zambezi, the real test of medical skills came at the rest camp.

Case history 12.1

Awakened in the middle of the night by a clinic nurse, I was presented to an African women in an obstructed stage of labour. Examination had to be made in candle light and the nearest technical means of delivery were two hours away. The ambulance transport had never been known to make the journey involved without breakdown. With mother and baby at risk I decided on a mad dash to the maternity clinic. In the dark, our transport all but collided with a truck which had struck a buffalo. The animal had died in the assault but the vehicle was thrown on its side to the decided detriment of the driver and his mate. The long suffering mother-to-be was joined by the two injured who were patched up as the journey continued and the poor woman laboured on.

At the clinic the promised baby life-saving equipment proved to be a very ancient ventouse extractor which was operated with the aid of a bicycle pump. The oedematous caput did not take kindly to the application of the bell extractor and a vacuum proved almost impossible to contrive. However, after several ineffective attempts, much to the relief of doctor, mother and baby the delivery was accomplished. With the cord tightly wrapped round the neck, the obstetric drama continued. Resuscitation was fraught with tension until the first spluttering inhalation relieved the stress on an anguished expedition medic. It was only then I recalled that 20 years had passed since my last personally conducted delivery. A brief obstetrics revision course might not be out of order for those about to accompany adventurers intent on visits to far-away places!

Choice of travel group

Elderly travellers

Avoid at all costs accompanying elderly devotees on tours specially designed for them, with a suicidal urge to embark on a holiday of a life-time to the end of the earth. These old-timers carry their chronic disorders with them and are always accompanied by suit-cases full of medicaments. Grounded by gout and arthritis, deterred by dyspnoea and congestion, few are fit enough to view the sights of global travel. They seek recompense by monopolising the attention of the captive tour doctor to his/her great discomfort.

Learn to distrust also the travel-hardened elder intent on 'do or die' trips to Mongolia or Alaska. The latter eventuality is all too likely with exposure to cold precipitating hypothermia or stroke. Exclude too, those contemplating post-retirement journeys to Machu Picchu, Kathmandu or Lhasa for en route they will succumb to pulmonary oedema or myocardial ischaemia and defy resuscitation. Casualty evacuation may mean carriage on a porter's back and be measured in days of walk rather than minutes by ambulance. Cross-border cadaver transfer is invariably fraught with anguish for the medical escort and may mean wearisome hours in transit while performing the last professional service to the departed.

Sudden deaths do little to enhance that important ingredient of the holiday package - the holiday spirit. This spirit can, however, be experienced to excess in younger groups where over-indulgence in cheap, potent, local libations brings maudlin merriment, self-inflicted injury, drunken coma and resultant inconvenience to the harassed group medic.

It is better to eschew well-publicised jaunts to conquer K4 or climb to some inaccessible summit in Bhutan. The 'tigers' of the high tops frequently peel off the mountain at a moment of maximal discomfort for the expedition doctor. Rendering first aid where exposure is both vertical and climatic, is not without hazard. Simple school trips to Gwent or Tangier must also be viewed with misgiving, for youngsters start vomiting the moment the boat leaves harbour, if not before. Their misguided antics result in bruises, breaks and blood-letting which will exasperate the medical companion.

Middle-aged travellers

Better by far to choose a group of the middle-aged in robust good health. Long separated from the boisterous over-activity of youth, they should be immune to the desire to climb impossible peaks. They tend to seek only creature comforts and a modicum of culture in a distant sunny clime. They never wander very far from life's simpler pleasures such as hot baths, flushing loos and good cuisine. Sadly such idyllic holidays involving butterfly-hunting in the Bahamas or shell-collecting in the Seychelles seem to elude me and offers of cave exploration in the Dordogne, a school trip to Boulogne or a pilgrimage to Lourdes never quite meet my expectations. The possibility of accompanying a hadj to Mecca was admittedly tempting, until study of the small print in the advertisement revealed the need for circumcision and conversion to Islam.

Young travellers

Sun, sand and sea were minimal prerequisites for my first working vacation and, misled by enticing travel brochures extolling the delights of the Land of the Midnight Sun, I signed up for the 'Lofoten lark'. This involved the medical care of 100 lads and lassies committed to exploration of the Arctic islands off north Norway. With the promise of 24 hours of daily sunshine I carefully packed adequate sun-screens and plenty of paperbacks for long days of leisure, free from the hassles of general medical practice.

Assured that I was joining a healthy bunch of teenagers, so they proved to be until the coastal steamer left the benevolent support of mainland medical facilities, and headed into the open Arctic Ocean. The burden of total medical care for the lusty one hundred began to weigh heavily upon me. With the Arctic circle and continental Norway hull-down beyond the horizon the first patients appeared as the ship wallowed and rolled in the Arctic swell, and sea-sickness began to take its toll.

Case history 12.1

Concealed within the vomiting horde, a medical trap for the unwary, was one girl whose emesis coincided with increasing pain in the right iliac fossa and rebound tenderness. Her condition quickly deteriorated as we plunged further into the Arctic wastes. An on-board pathologist took a morbid interest in my diagnosis, and a fiendish delight in listing the dangers of delayed surgical intervention, I feverishly considered the inadequacy of our first-aid pack for emergency appendicectomy. Lacking the courage to put rusty surgical skills to the test I opted for procrastination and sweated out the crossing to the Lofoten Islands, wondering if my defence society subscriptions were up-to-date and their cover world-wide. At the first port of call the patient was whisked by land-rover to a tiny operating unit where she was promptly relieved of an evil-looking appendix.

Secure in the belief that the surgical drama of the expedition now lay behind us, small groups set off to storm the mighty Lofoten 'Wall' and battle south to the

Maelstrom or the outermost parts of the island chain. By boat, ferry, dirt track and mountain trail, they struck out across fiord and loch, bog and boulders, screes and sands. One party camped at the most western point of Arctic Norway.

Case history 13.2

In splendid solitude, far from human habitation, a lad suddenly developed an acute abdomen.

An hour's boat trip over storm-tossed waters and another hour's trudge over precipitous slopes separated doctor and patient. By the time we met, the diagnosis of another acute appendix was not in doubt. A launch trip across waves of Arctic proportions did little to settle the intestinal inflammation; nor did the overland ride. We lurched along rough tracks in a mad race to catch inter-island ferries in a long nail-biting run up the archipelago to the welcome haven of a village hospital and another urgent appendicectomy operation. The prolonged evacuation provoked an anxiety which robbed me of much of the tranquillity engendered by a sojourn in this remote Arctic wilderness.

Himalayan travels

One can indeed pay a heavy price in stress and strain in return for the advantages of free travel. Slow to learn from experience, I next set out with a stalwart climbing party, intent on answering the 'call of Kolahoi', a formidable 6,000m Himalayan mountain in Kashmir. This time the first-aid gear provided for emergency surgery and large containers were painfully lugged over high mountain passes. Most of the contents remained untouched during the trip.

A few days into the trek, along dry, dusty sun-parched tracks, the party plunged themselves into a stream spilling from a mountain chasm. Canteens and bellies were filled appreciatively with water until the decomposing body of

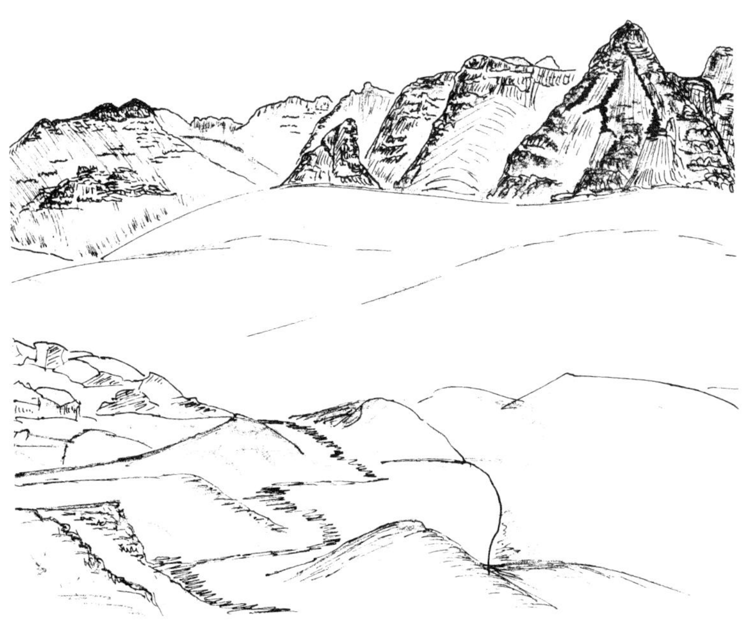

an Indian woman was discovered a few yards upstream. The potential onslaught of some dread disease was a constant companion over the ensuing days of trek. Each bout of the inevitable travellers' diarrhoea was viewed with foreboding.

Decompression sickness

No one succumbed, although bed-bugs left remarkable evidence of their nocturnal feasts on party members. They preferred the soft-skinned women climbers, whereas fleas of Himalayan stature afflicted male mountaineers. Kashmir 'collywobbles' struck indiscriminately. A mere inconvenience at lower altitudes, a bared posterior high on an exposed mountain risks frost-nip in intimate places. Enteritis, however, ceased to be a problem when the expedition ran out of food three days and 3,000m above the re-supply point.

Acute mountain sickness (AMS), always a threat at high altitude, is no respecter of persons. On this trip, the only one affected was my medical colleague.

Case history 12.3

He developed cerebral manifestations of altitude sickness which divorced him from reality. Our climbing status was badly dented when he had to be physically restrained from making a solo ascent up a fearsome nearby mountain after he developed hallucinations and delusions. His behaviour was quite irrational and he nearly lost his life when leaving the tent in the middle of the night and walking off alone across the glacier. Only benign weather conditions allowed us to reach him before he fell into a crevasse. Our reputation took another knock by my spectacular 100m fall down the snout of the Kolohoi glacier. A flailing ice-axe nicked a new dimple in my chin and the expedition all but lost its medical cover.

Casualty skills came in useful back at base camp. A pressure cooker blew up. Lid and contents made a very big hole in the tent, and a slightly smaller one in the cook who was bending over the appliance at the time. It proved difficult, in treatment, to separate the stew from part-boiled brown Indian flesh.

Leaving the dubious delights of Kashmir behind, we hastened to Delhi, promptly discarded all the first-aid impediments, and took the bus for Agra.

Case history 12.4

The leader shortly after became acutely ill with symptoms which necessitated examination and conference by the combined expedition medical fraternity. Prostrated across the back seat of the vehicle, he was little reassured by the earnest case consultation his condition precipitated. A gynaecologist, bacteriologist, GP and a physician, all intent on seeing the Taj

Mahal, gave it as their considered opinion that he was fit for onward travel!

Once at Agra a temporary improvement in his malaise allowed us to lay him out on the emerald green lawns of the magnificent Taj. He was then deserted by his medical guardians who went off to marvel at the many splendours of the Mogul shrines. He was afterwards escorted back to Delhi and hustled on to a UK bound jet with solace from solicitous stewardesses. He made an uneventful return to his home in the Western Isles and a much more eventful ambulance flight to Glasgow a day or two later to have a laparotomy and cholecystectomy. Slightly disturbed by this turn of events, we reminded ourselves that our first duty as his medical advisers was to keep him clear of the mud-floored, jam-packed and often unhygienic hospitals of rural India, and that our inactivity had ensured his survival - just!

Asia Minor

By now a committed expeditioner, the next trip took me to Asia Minor and the torrid, desolate wastes of the Taurus mountains. Disaster nearly occurred en route for the coach driver, high on drugs and drink, would insist on driving without hands on the steering wheel. The situation became more serious when he attempted to steer with his feet. The nadir of the journey was reached when the coach glanced off an on-coming car to the decided disadvantage of the latter. Tempers frayed and knives were drawn in the ensuing driver-to-driver confrontation which became desparate when the Turkish police finally arrived. As neither driver had insurance and only one had a licence, the initial police intent was to imprison all involved, offenders and on-lookers. Suitably chastened and with a new driver, we were ultimately allowed to continue on our way.

Once into the waterless mountains, sunburn, dehydration and Turkey trots made pressing demands on the medics. High up on the mountain plateau, tough nomads live in black hessian tents with open fires, and all our dressings went on children hideously burnt and with nasty, suppurating, chronic wounds.

East Africa

The medical bags were next packed for East Africa and ascents of Kilimanjaro and Mount Kenya. Iatrogenic illness struck early when one expedition doctor turned a not unbecoming, if rather alarming, shade of blue. The anti-malarial prophylactic had prepared his blood more for the company of the Blue Men of the Sahara rather than the snows of Kilimanjaro.

On this trip at last, our surgical skills were finally put to use. As guests of honour at an African durbar, we were presented with a sword for the ceremonial slaughter of two sheep. Knowledge of the arterial supply certainly expedited the blood-letting. Many of the party were to later suffer from the indiscreet consumption of black puddings made from the collected blood and entrails of the unfortunate animals. No longer does counting sheep ease me into slumber. I always recall the anguished eyes of the sacrificed beasts prior to death, a reproach retained beyond their demise as they were later offered as delicacies at the feast.

Kilimanjaro, at 6,300 metres altitude, induces acute mountain sickness and the night climb to the summit is psychologically daunting. Climbers with dyspnoea, vomiting and headaches kept doctors busy. Mount Kenya brought fewer problems but there it seemed that I had been finally overtaken by AMS. Awakened by bizarre undulations under my sleeping bag in the small hours I searched the tent in vain for intruders. Awakened later by a similar disturbance, I flexed my legs and thumped them down upon the ground. All became still and blaming hallucinations I returned to sleep. In the morning a large fur-eared mountain rat lay dead beneath the sleeping bag and a two foot hole in the ground sheet and the tent was testimony to his night-time activities.

Our high climbers, in snow on the equator, suffered from AMS, developed cerebral and pulmonary manifestations of the disease, and became overdue. An initial air search did not find them and the delay was psychologically traumatic for the waiting doctors. A measure of anxiety still prevailed on return to the UK.

'Doctor will travel'

A long-suffering wife therafter, prohibited distant medical travel and the next vacation was spent doing DIY jobs at home. Having safely negotiated the highest peaks in Africa and Europe, I thereupon fell 10 metres from the gable of the house to land on top of ladder, scaffold and wife in that order. With great forbearance the lady, injured in body and mind, promptly recommended far-distant pastures for further holiday exploits.

Once again I scan the situation vacant columns, Expedition medic required.' 'Doctor will travel', I reply.

Appendix I

Dangers from the sun while abroad

Over exposure to the sun can not only bring severe sunburn but it also brings a risk of heat stroke, dehydration and cancer of the skin.

The further south towards the equator the holiday venue the greater the effect of the sun's rays, eg. in Southern Spain the sun's rays are twice as harmful as in the UK.

Adverse effects from the sun are greatest between 10 am and 3 pm.

Graded exposure for a short time in half hour intervals is a wise precaution to avoid adverse effects of the sun.

High reflection on the beach by the waterside also increases the sun's effects, and rays can pass through lightly woven material such as thin shirts and blouses. Adequate protection from the sun's rays can only be obtained from protective sun screen lotions and creams using the highest factors - above 10 and up to 15. These should be applied and frequently reapplied on all children and fair skinned adults.

Skin cancer is a serious risk to fair skinned, blue-eyed, red and fair haired people who freckle. The effects of the rays build up with continued exposure over the years. The risk can only be decreased by avoiding direct exposure to sunlight from 10 am to 3 pm and by adequate coverage with the highest factor protective sun creams at other times. Sun worshippers must remember that the sun can kill and limit exposure to dangerous rays.

Cloud cover may be misleading. The warming sensation of heat is decreased and people stay out in shaded sunlight for longer. Ultra violet light rays pass through light cloud cover and can still burn.

Surface ultra-violet light reflection can cause problems as sand reflects a quarter of light rays and three quarters of the rays will be transmitted through water to affect the swimmer.

The higher the sun in the sky, the shorter the ray-path and the greater the risk of skin burning.

Appendix II

Vaccinations and malaria prevention

People return regularly from holiday and develop **malaria** which can be fatal. Increased resistance to drug therapy means that many people are inadequately protected.

Over much of **Asia, India, Africa and South America** there is a high risk of malaria infection. Travellers to these areas should start appropriate medication one week prior to departure on holiday and continue for six weeks after their return.

Active prevention

Mosquitoes are the source of malaria infection and it cannot be assumed that taking drugs is sufficient to protect the individual.

Long trousers, long sleeved shirts and blouses should be worn for protection if bites are to be avoided. Exposed areas of the face, hands and neck should be covered with preparations such as DEET or Jungle Formula which can be bought from the chemist.

Hotel rooms should be sprayed with appropriate anti-mosquito repellents or a pyrrethrum coil should be ignited to deter the insects.

Even transient visits of an hour or two to infected areas, can result in infection. People in transit stops on air journeys have been infected at airports.

Vaccination against other diseases

Cholera and typhoid, hepatitis and AIDS are common in many parts of the world. All travellers who live in the UK should ensure that they have been vaccinated against polio and tetanus. If there is a risk of cholera, typhoid, yellow fever or hepatitis, they should also have the appropriate vaccination.

Random sexual encounters in Asia and Africa have a high riks of infection with **HIV** and the later development of **AIDS** disease. The use of condom protection decreases the risk but does not wholly protect against infection. In the absence of a cure, avoidance is the only certain means of protection.

Dental needles, chiropody instruments and injections can transmit disease in parts of Asia and Africa, and treatment should be avoided if at all possible while overseas.

Appendix III

Contaminated water spreads disease when abroad

Contaminated water is a very frequent source of diarrhoeal illness in travellers. Outwith Western Europe and North America the water is nearly always suspect, and along the shores of the Mediterranean it may also be contaminated.

When travelling it is best to assume that water supplies harbour disease. Hotel tap water should be sterilised with puritabs and in the Tropics, Asia and Africa, sterilised water should even be used for cleaning teeth.

WATER CAN BE STERILISED BY ADDING PURITABS (BOUGHT FROM ANY CHEMIST) AND WILL BE FIT FOR CONSUMPTION WITHIN HALF AN HOUR OF TREATMENT.

The iodine taste can be disguised by the addition of orange powder.

WATER CAN ALSO BE STERILISED BY BOILING AND USE OF A TRAVELLERS KETTLE OR ELECTRIC COIL can be a convenience when travelling abroad.

Ice for drinks is a frequent source of diarrhoeal infection and the addition of ice cubes should be avoided. Ideally, one should drink from commercially bottled water or carbonated water in foreign parts but in some countries such as India and China, even the commercial supplies may be contaminated.

Diarrhoeal and vomiting illness which comes with infection when abroad, requires treatment by fluid replacement and this requires copious input of fluids in small amounts.

If diarrhoea and vomiting occur the best solution is to use bottles of flat coke or carbonated drinks. The necks of bottles or the tops of tins of commercial drinks also carry disease and they should be cleaned with wet, medicated wipes before being used as drinking receptacles.

It is a wise precaution to carry a packet of drinking straws on global journeys. Used to sip drinks, they reduce risk of infection from contaminated bottle tops or cups.

Fruit and vegetables are often washed in contaminated water abroad, and salads are should be avoided if the water source is suspect.

Appendix IV

INFECTED FOOD CAN CAUSE DISEASE

Diarrhoeal illness is very common in travellers and can spoil the holiday.

Diarrhoeal illness is avoidable with precautions.

Most traveller's diarrhoea results from swallowing contaminated food and drink.

Diarrhoeal illness is usually self-limiting and will get better after one to three days with no treatment other than replacement of body water losses.

Hints on safe eating and drinking abroad

Food choice:

Choose food that must have been freshly cooked, eg, omelettes or chips.

Freshly boiled food is always safe eg. rice.

Peel all fruit and vegetables before eating.

Eat food from sealed packs or cans.

Do not eat: salads, shellfish, unpeeled fruit or vegetables, ice-cream and ices.

Sauces and relishes left out on the table or food on which insects have settled will be infected.

Remember, contaminated plates and cutlery not washed with detergent or rinsed in clean water and protected from flies, can cause infection

Hands and fingers should be washed at every opportunity, preferably in water with added disinfectant.

Only eat food that you have handled if your hands are scrupulously clean.

Drinking water

Outwith Western Europe and North America, drinking water is nearly always suspect and should be boiled before use or sterilised with puritabs.

Ice is often frozen, contaminated water. Ice cubes and iced drinks spread disease.

If in doubt, if food is not cooked, boiled or peeled, avoid it.

Index

A

abdominal surgery 106
abortion 96
acclimatisation 150
acetazolamide 84, 152 - 153
actinic keratosis 113
actinic rays 94
acute mountain sickness 145 - 146, 149, 165, 167
adventure travel 88
agoraphobia 49 - 50, 55,56
AIDS xv, 81, 91, 138, 158, 172
air embolism 137
air travel 36, 48, 55, 60, 87, 95, 97, 102, 105, 117,123,126
algal bloom 83, 132, 139,141
d-amphetamine 69
AMS 146 - 148, 150, 152 - 155, 158, 165, 167 - 168
  fatal 147
  signs and symptoms 151
anaemia 96, 106
angina 111, 153
anoxia 42,148
anti-HAV titres 27
anti-malarials 76
anticholinergics 24
anxiety 36 - 37, 42, 49, 55 - 56, 168
  overt 52
anxyolitics 94
appendicectomy 162
Arctic hysteria 42
area postrema 65
ascending pyelonephritis 91
aseptic meningitis 133
assessing the risk 11
asthmatics 22,138
ataxia 152
attack rate ix
automonic response 66
avoidable deaths 131
avoidance behaviour 46-47

B

baby feeding 75
back-packers xv,xvi, 23,158
barotrauma 137
behaviour therapy 44, 56, 94
Benzodiazepines 45, 55
bilharzia 82 - 83, 91, 132 - 133, 143
bites
  insects 83
  scorpions 83
  snakes 83
blind travellers 124
blue-green algae 132
body clock 40
bowel disorder 23
breast feeding 75

C

calf muscle cramps 96
car-sickness 66, 71
  management 70

cardiovascular illness 104-106
categories of handicap 122
cercarial dermatitis 134
cerebral arterial insufficiency 111
cerebral oedema 151
cerebrovascular accident 105-106
child traveller 73, 77
    high altitude 84
    immunization 76
    management 75
    planning 74
    pressure changes 75
chloroquine 99
cholera 5, 8 - 9, 33, 76, 172
chronic obstructive
    airways disease 20
cinnarizine 78
circadian rhythm 2, 20, 22, 38 - 40, 42, 81, 90
circulatory disturbance 63
coach travel 126
coelenterates 135
Communicable Disease Unit (CDSU) viii
conditioned response 47
confused elderly 106
congestive heart failure xviii
conjunctivitis 83, 132
contaminated feeds 75
contaminated water 173
continence 129
contractual assessment 20
corals 135, 143
coronary bypass surgery 153
cruising holidays 113
cultural shock 40
current risk status 19
cyano bacteria 132
cyclizine 69
cylinder oxygen 148

D

dangerous fish 134
database 4
decompression sickness 136 - 137, 143, 164
defects
    hearing 129
    limb deformity 129
    mental faculty 129
    sight 129
dehydration 64, 112, 141
dementia 106
dependent oedema 96
depressed patients 39
depressive state 50
desensitisation 21, 56 - 57, 59 - 60, 94
dexamethasone 152
diabetic 22
diabetic medication] 109
diabetic neuropathy 24
diabetics 110
diarrhoea 80, 104
diarrhoeal disease 10
diarrhoeal illness 174 - 175
dioralyte 80
diphtheria xvi, 76
the disabled 2, 106, 120
    management 125
disabled rail travellers 127
disabled traveller
    management 129
disabled travellers 121 - 123
disproportionate fear 51
disturbances
    metabolism 2
diuretic therapy 107
diuretics xviii
diver 137
diving hazards 131, 135, 136
douching
    rectal 140
    vaginal 140
drinking water 176
drowning 131,134, 135, 141, 143
drug abuse 29, 31, 44
drug resistance xvii
drug therapy 13,20, 22, 67
dysentery 24
dyspnoea 111

E

ear infection 62,63,132
early women travellers 86
elation 40
the elderly traveller 101, 109, 148, 160
effects of travel 105
management 117
electrolyte imbalance 64
emergency transportation 14
emetic process 65
enteric-transmitted
non-A non-B hepatitis 98
environmental change 42
environmental stress36
erythema 135
establishing the clinic 4
euphoria 40
eustachian problems75
excluded travellers 41, 106
expedition medicine 157
extremes of temperature and
altitude 111

F

factors affecting travellers
health xii
fatal AMS 147
fatigue 139
fear of
enclosed spaces 50
needles 54
fears and phobias 41, 52
fee schedule 6
female condom 93
female phobics 50
Femidom 93
first aid kit xviii, 31, 158
fish bites 143
flooding 57, 59
fluid retention 150
flying phobias 47 - 48, 56
foreign body penetration 143
fractures
cervical spine 138
skull 138
FREMEC 123
Freudian approach 53
the functionally disabled 21

G

gall-bladder disease 104
gamma globulin 80, 84
gas embolism 138
gastro-enteritis 104
gastrointestinal haemorrhage 106
graded exposure 169
gravel burns 143
gross peripherial oedema 109
group travel 41 - 42
groupers 134
Growth in international travel ix
guide dogs 124

H

H_2 blockers 24
HACO 151
haematological reserve 105
haematuria 91, 141
hallucinate 58
handicapped traveller 12, 129
HAPO151
HAV 26 - 27, 31
Havrix 27, 28, 81
hazards of land travel 43
hazards of watersports 134
HBV transmission 28, 29
health counsellor 2
health hazards 131
health promotion 1, 2, 5
heart disease 153
heat-stroke 112
hepatitis 33, 158, 172
hepatitis A 5, xi, xvi, 24 - 25, 27 - 28, 31 - 32, 34, 76, 80 - 81, 98
fulminant hepatitis A
infection 25
risk 26
symptoms 25
hepatitis A vaccine 9

hepatitis B 25, 28, 81
high altitude 16, 145, 149, 155
high altitude climbing 155
high altitude disease146, 151
high risk group 11 - 12
high-factor sun screens 82
HIV 13, 29, 31, 33, 93, 97, 138, 172
homosexual 29
hookworm 83, 141
hormonal contraception 92
1-Hyoscine 68 - 69
    patch 68
    side-effects 68
hypertension 153
hyperthermia 158
hyperventilation 63, 135,143, 150
hypnotherapy 44, 57, 59 - 60
hypocapnia 63
hypomania 38
hypothermia 84, 131, 134, 136, 139, 143, 158
hypoxia 42, 105, 149, 151

I

IATA 123
iatrogenic illness 167
ice for drinks 173, 176
ill effects on the confused 109
immune deficiencies 24
immune response xi
Immunisation 9
immunoglobulin 27, 98
implosion 57
imprisonment 89
in-flight immobility 108
inadequate medical care 110
Inca trail 42
increased red cell production 150
infected food 175
infections 2
    cyano bacterial 143
    gastroenteritis 143
    hepatitis 143
    HIV 143
    leptospirosis 143
infectious diarrhoea 24
infective hepatitis xv
insect bites xvii, 158
insulin 110, 129
insurance cover xiv, 2, 104, 110
international travel 74
intestinal disorder 104
intrauterine growth 96
intravenous therapy 91
irrational fear51

J

Japan 9
jelly fish stings 143
jet-lag 2, 40, 45, 81, 113, 129

L

Larva migransi 83, 143
leech bites 143
leeches 91, 93
    aquatic 135
leg exercises 92
leptospirosis 83, 132 - 133, 141
lesions113
limb deformities 124
listeriosis 97

M

major chest surgery 106
malaria vii, xiii, xvi, 1, 93, 171
malignant change 113
Malignant falciparum malaria xi
malignant melanoma 82, 94
management protocol 4
MASTA xiii, xv
mediastinal emphysema 137
MEDIF 123
menorrhagia 89, 90
mental confusion 42
the mentally unstable 39
modelling
    participant 56
    vicarious 56, 59

modes of transport 35
monilial infection 91
morbid depression 42
mosquitoes 93, 141
motion sickness 2, 21, 62, 64 - 65
mountaineers 145, 148, 164
myocardial infarction 106
myocardial ischaemia 153
myoglobinuria 141

N

neoplastic skin change 94
nitrogen narcosis 135

O

off-shore winds 134
the old 2
oral contraceptives 69, 90, 153
organising the database 4
orthopaedic emergency xiv

P

package holidays vii, 2
panic reaction 49
paranoia 40
pelvic inflammatory disease 143
peripheral oedema 92
pertussis 76
pharmacological blocking agents 65
phase retardation 39
phobia2, 51, 53, 94
    flying 56, 59
    management 55
    medication 55
    therapy 54
physical handicap 121, 122
placenta separation 96
PMS 92
pneumonia 83, 139, 141
pneumothorax 137 - 138
poliomyelitis xi,5, 8, 9, 76, 98, 172
polycythaemia 150
pooling 63
post-hypnotic suggestions 58 - 59
postural hypotension 63
pre-existing disease 12,17, 20, 22,104
pre-flight anxieties 36
pre-travel consultation 7, 74
pregnancy 2, 94 - 98, 138, 148
    medical management 99
    preparing for travel 97
premature labour 94, 96
premenstrual syndrome 90
primary care resources 20,105
prochlorperazine syrup 78
proguanil 99
Promethazine 69, 76
prophylaxis 2, vii, 19
psychological distress 21, 63, 85, 87,104, 106
pulmonary problems 109, 123, 137, 150
puritabs 173

Q

quarantine 124
questionnaire 10, 17

R

rabid dogs 83
random sexual encounters 172
Rapture of the Deep 136
rat urine 132, 141
red-backed spider bite 91
reflexes
    fight 52
    regular medication 107
rehydrat 80
relaxation 53
relocation 76
rescues 147
respiratory 63,105,150, 153
risk 19 - 20
    identified 2
    quantified 2
risk assessment viii

rota virus 80
rotational stimulation 65

S

S mansoni 133
sail-board problems 138
Salmonella 24,80
salpingitis 140
sand-flies 93, 141
sand-worm infestation xvii
schistosome larvae 134
schistosomiasis 133
scopoderm patches 21
Scopolamine 68
scuba divers 137
sea travel 126
sea urchin spines 139, 143
sea-sickness 71, 87, 162
season 20
secondary amenorrhoa 89
senescence 115
sexually promiscuous 31
sexually transmitted disease 93
skeletal injury 143
skin cancer 169
sky chair 107
the sleep-wake cycle 42, 89
small boat risks 141
spasticity 129
special risk travellers 106
spinal cord injuries 140
spontaneous abortion 95
sports-induced infections 131
standardised questionnaire 17
stasis oedema 92
sterilising water 173
stingrays 134
stress 35 - 36, 44, 66, 129, 150
  cardiac 145
  management 44
  pulmonary 145
stress tolerance threshold 36
stressors 37
sub aqua 135
sun-blocks 94, 113, 169
sunburn 82,142 - 143, 169
surfing accidents 131
surfing problems 138
swimmers' itch 134
swimming pools 132
syncope 63

T

tears
  rectal 140
  vaginal 140
tetanus 5, 8, 9, 76, 98, 172
tetraplegia 138
therapeutic abortion 90
thermal regulation 2
thrombosis 109, 123
time zone crossing
  insulin 111
  routines 45, 113
  transition 40 , 76
tissue infestation 143
toxaemia 96
train transportation 127
Transatlantic crossings vii
transdermal patch 68 - 71
transfusion 91
transmedian flights 42, 45
transmeridian disturbances 38
transportation-induced stress viii
trauma 2
trauma infection 158
traumatic peritonitis 96
TRAVAX xviii
travel agents xi
travel health clinic 1 - 2, 5, vii, 20, 60, 120, 122, 125
travel insurance 15
  limitations 94
travel phobia 21, 47, 94
travel sickness 62, 66, 77, 158
  automomic symptoms 63
  cause 64
  habituation 65
  instructions for parents 79
  prevention 66
  significant problems 63
  variability of symptoms 64

travel-induced disease viii
travel-induced illness viii, ix,1- 2, 7, 10, 17, 74, 105
traveller's death x
travellers' diarrhoea 23, 79
travelling with children 78
treatment
  acupuncture 31
  chiropody 31
  dental 31
trekkers 145, 147 - 148, 150
tsetse flies 93
typhoid 5, 9, xi, 33, 76, 172

U

ulcers 135
urinary tract infections 90-91
UTI 91

V

vaccination 1, 7 - 8, x, xii - xiii, 19, 28, 76, 81, 84, 97 - 98, 126, 129, 148, 158, 171 - 172
  diphtheria 98
  hepatitis A 98
  hepatitis B 98
  Japanese encephalitis xvii
  meningococcal polysaccharide 98
  package xi
  pre-travel 55
  rabies xvii, 98
  tetanus 98
  travel 33
  typhoid xvi
  vivotif 33
vaginal infection 93
vaginal lacerations 96
variables
  biochemical 40
  physiological 40
  psychological 40
vector-borne disease 92, 113,133
venereal infection 93
venous thrombosis 96 - 97
very frail old 20
vestibular stimulation 67
vulval lacerations 96

W

water sports 131
  health hazards 143
water-skiing 139
weals 135
wheelchair 107, 125, 127
windsurfers 138, 139
the woman traveller 86
  risks 89

Y

Yellow fever xvi, 76, 172
yellow fever vaccine 9
the young 2
young travellers 161

Z

Zeitbergers 40